Sleep Easy with Natural Methods

Simple, science-backed ways to restful sleep.
No pills, No gimmicks. Easy to follow sleep tips.

I0102287

Venkata L Buddharaju MD
Board Certified Sleep Physician

Sleep Easy with Natural Methods

ISBN: 978-0-635-44616-9

About the Author

Dr. Venkata L Buddharaju (or Dr. Buddha, as his patients call him) is a fellowship-trained physician at the Albany Medical Center in Albany, New York. He is Board Certified in Internal Medicine, Pulmonary, Critical Care, and Sleep Medicine by the American Board of Internal Medicine. He now teaches and consults at hospital intensive care units and pulmonary units, as well as sleep medical practices.

He directs the Sleep Disorders Center and Clinic at Thorek Memorial Hospital in Chicago. In addition to treating other sleep disorders, for over at least two decades, Dr. Buddharaju has counseled natural methods and improved the sleep of many of his patients.

Dr. Buddharaju has numerous medical-device patents and is working to develop more patient-friendly medical devices. Throughout his career, he has conducted clinical research, published his work in various medical journals, and worked to develop and implement high-quality patient-care policies. He believes strongly that balancing natural healing practices with traditional medicine is important for the future of effective healthcare.

Table of Contents

About the Author ii

Special Thanks v

Dedication vi

INTRODUCTION ix

Preface... xiv

SECTION 1...1

Chapter 1 Sleep Basics...2

Section 2: Common Sleep Problems: 17

Chapter 2 Sleep Disorders 18

Section 3: Natural Methods for Sleep.........................24

Chapter 3 Exercise and Sleep 25

Chapter 4 Diet and Sleep 36

Chapter 5 Stress and Sleep.......................................47

Chapter 6 A Word About Sleep Hygiene 70

Chapter 7 Time Management and Sleep......................77

Chapter 8 Music and Sleep 84

Chapter 9 Nature and Sleep 88

Epilogue 93

Appendix Good Sleep Hygiene Practices....................95

Bibliography and Suggested Reading.........................100

Sleep Tips...104

Special Thanks

To my wife, Srilatha Buddharaju, without whom so much, including this book, would not be possible. She has supported me in every endeavor and sacrificed her time to raise our sons, Anudeep Buddharaju (a lawyer) and Sandeep Buddharaju (a doctor), with compassion, and instilled in them the courage to deal with the world.

Dedication

To my late father, B.V. Bangarraju, whose guidance at every step of my life shaped me into who I am today. And to my mother, B. Satyavathi, whose love and compassion continue to inspire me to help others.

Human Life

"We live nine months as a fetus, sleep most of the time as a baby, and spend a third of our adult life asleep. Time is precious. Use it wisely."

—Venkata L Buddharaju

INTRODUCTION

Growing up in India from the 1970s to 1990s, people didn't stay up late at night. We ate dinner as a family, went to bed when sleepy, and awoke naturally at sunrise. My mom used to say that the best time to read and study was early morning, when the mind was calm and the world hadn't woken up yet. We socialized almost daily, and no one talked about sleep issues at home or in a doctor's office.

I was surprised to find a different lifestyle when I came to the United States in 1992 for internal, pulmonary, critical care, and sleep medicine education. I have been practicing medicine in Chicago for more than twenty years now. I work longer hours and struggle to balance work and family, sacrificing my creative time.

Sleep is a basic human need, but we live in a high-stress society where work, family, and financial demands don't allow us enough time to relax and spend quality time together. Many of my patients and colleagues have experienced sleep struggles ranging from minor sleep difficulties to severe insomnia, snoring, sleep apnea, and more.

Over the decades, humans have gradually reduced the time they spend in quality sleep and are awake longer in a twenty-four-hour cycle. According to a study by the Centers for Disease Control and Prevention (CDC) and other studies, about 35 percent of US adults are not getting the recommended seven to nine hours of sleep on a regular basis. Even teenagers, who need extra hours of sleep (eight to ten hours), are spending less time sleeping. According to a 2006 National Sleep Foundation poll, 87 percent of US high school students get far less than the recommended eight to ten hours of sleep.

Some of the consequences of poor sleep are anxiety, depression, suicidal thoughts, obesity, diabetes, hypertension, stroke, heart attack, excessive daytime sleepiness, poor concentration, and an increased risk for motor vehicle and other accidents. In addition to these worrisome health consequences and sleep deprivation's impact on the body and mind, America's lack of sleep is costing billions of healthcare dollars.

Humans live an average of sixty to eighty years, depending on where they live on the planet. People live much longer in some parts of the world than they do in others. The people of Okinawa, Japan, report one of the world's highest life expectancies. In general, across the world, human life expectancy has steadily increased with advances in infection control, technology, and medicine. However, one thing that has not changed is the medical community's recommendations for sleep time and duration.

We spend approximately 40 percent—a third of our lifetime—asleep, which we don't remember, except for occasional dreams. At sunset, our brain releases a chemical substance called melatonin, which makes us sleepy and helps us get into sleep mode. Wake-promoting hormones decline at this time of day, and sleep-promoting substances increase with the onset of sleep. Caffeine, alcohol, or other substances we consume can interfere with this balance and cause sleep difficulties such as insomnia and poor sleep quality.

Our brain clock, called the circadian rhythm, wakes us up at sunrise, bringing us to a conscious level so that we can function optimally throughout the day. The longer we are awake, the higher the concentration of adenosine, a sleep-promoting neurotransmitter that we need at the end of the day.

This sleep-wake cycle has evolved over thousands of years in various species, including humans. This cycle continues unabated unless interrupted intentionally by activity, diet, stress, or other health conditions.

A good night's sleep prior to a major performance—such as a musical concert, athletic match, important academic test, or corporate presentation—is key for optimal performance. A well-rested brain and body feel more positive and perform much better. On the other hand, students who stay up too late and sleep only a few hours prior to a major exam do poorly on the test due to their inability to focus. That's because the information learned during their awake state is stored in the memory centers of the brain during sleep, particularly in deep Rapid Eye Movement (REM) sleep, which is when most dreams occur. They have not given their brain enough sleep time to process the information they learned during the day. As a result, they do not retain the information.

According to a 2023 US Gallup poll survey, the majority of US adults (57%) say they would feel better if they got more sleep. Women have been less likely to get enough sleep than men. These trends represent significant declines in sleep from previous surveys in 2004 and 2013. A culture shift with rapid technological development is likely to blame. People live automatic, mechanical lives, spending increasingly more time on devices and looking into screens emitting blue light, even closer to bedtime. This hinders the release of melatonin from the brain's pituitary gland, an important neuro-hormone that helps us get to sleep. Those who sleep less also feel more stressed, and stress makes people sleep less. Thus, there is a positive correlation between lack of sleep and the level of stress in life.

Sleep is a natural process that has evolved over millions of years in all life forms; animals and humans are no exception. Long before the industrial revolution and the invention of light-emitting screens, televisions, computers, and technology, humans naturally woke up at sunrise and were active throughout the day, perhaps taking a nap late in the afternoon before going back to sleep at sunset when it was dark. Now we live in a 24/7 society with excess light exposure, even close to bedtime, so our brains are tricked into thinking it is still daytime. This shuts down the release of melatonin, which is required to naturally go to sleep. If we feel sleepy, we gulp coffee, sometimes stronger espresso, to suppress the natural sleep hormone adenosine, released from the basal forebrain, which counteracts adenosine and prevents us from falling asleep.

We try to go to bed with a ton of things on our minds that are still active, on top of consuming brain stimulants, and try to watch late-night TV, computers, and phone screens, scrolling social media hoping to fall asleep.

We live under the false belief that we can do anything and nothing will happen to us. Unfortunately, our brains are not wired that way but are meant to follow the natural rhythmic flow that has evolved over millions of years. We also don't seem to understand the need for enough sleep.

Over the years, I have counseled thousands of patients to improve their sleep habits for better sleep and to enhance their daytime function and productivity in whatever they do while awake. I have also interviewed people from diverse fields and identified a connection between sleep and happiness. As a result, I sought practical, natural methods to improve sleep and quality of life.

The vicious cycle of sleepless nights and daytime worry due to less than optimal performance makes things worse. The two feed one another. But, by making small changes to your lifestyle and eliminating distractions, you can open up the door for more focused attention. This will lead to increased productivity at work and more success at both work and home. These changes should bring needed sleep and a chance to live a happier life. Lifestyle modification involves removing distractions. I hope you will find the information in this book valuable and helpful in bringing about the necessary yet simple changes to get better sleep and lead a happier life and also be productive in whatever we do during our awake state.

Sleep is necessary for survival. However, humanity's solution to sleep problems is often medication. I am not a big fan of medications. In this book, I share some of the simple, natural solutions that can help address the sleep problems many face today. In addition to giving practical tips to improve sleep, I have also included at the end of each chapter at least two sleep habits that you seriously want to change and see if you sleep better and feel better the next morning. I want to hear from you as a reader of this book so that we can make a difference together in the lives of people.

I formatted this revised book with a new title, Sleep Easy with Natural Methods, and divided it into three sections. Section 1 covers the basic fundamentals of sleep, explaining what happens to our brain and body during sleep, how much sleep we need, what neurochemical hormones play a role in promoting sleep and wake states, and how the natural circadian clock works and maintains a natural rhythm of sleep. In Section 2, I will discuss common sleep conditions. In Section 3, I will discuss in detail how one can improve their sleep by following natural methods, including a daily routine to maintain a natural rhythm of regular sleep-wake, exercise, sleep-promoting diet, avoiding habits that keep you awake (like light exposure, caffeine, and other stimulants), how to wind down a restless mind, and finally, incorporating nature walks and music. At the end of each chapter in Section 3, I would like you to try two new sleep habits for two to four weeks and see if that helps you sleep better and feel better in the morning so that you can incorporate them into your daily routine.

Venkata L Buddharaju, MD, FCCP, FAASM
Board Certified Internal Medicine, Pulmonary,
Critical Care and Sleep Medicine.

Preface

Of the Better Sleep Happier Life

With increasing awareness of sleep for health and happiness, and advances in understanding of how sleep affects our health, I have decided to edit my first edition of my book and add a new chapter called "Tips for Better Sleep" by adopting some easy-to-follow habits.

The main chapters remain the same with some additional information added based on recent updates since the original publication in April 2020. That was right around the time of the COVID pandemic, which devastated millions of people's lives and sleep.

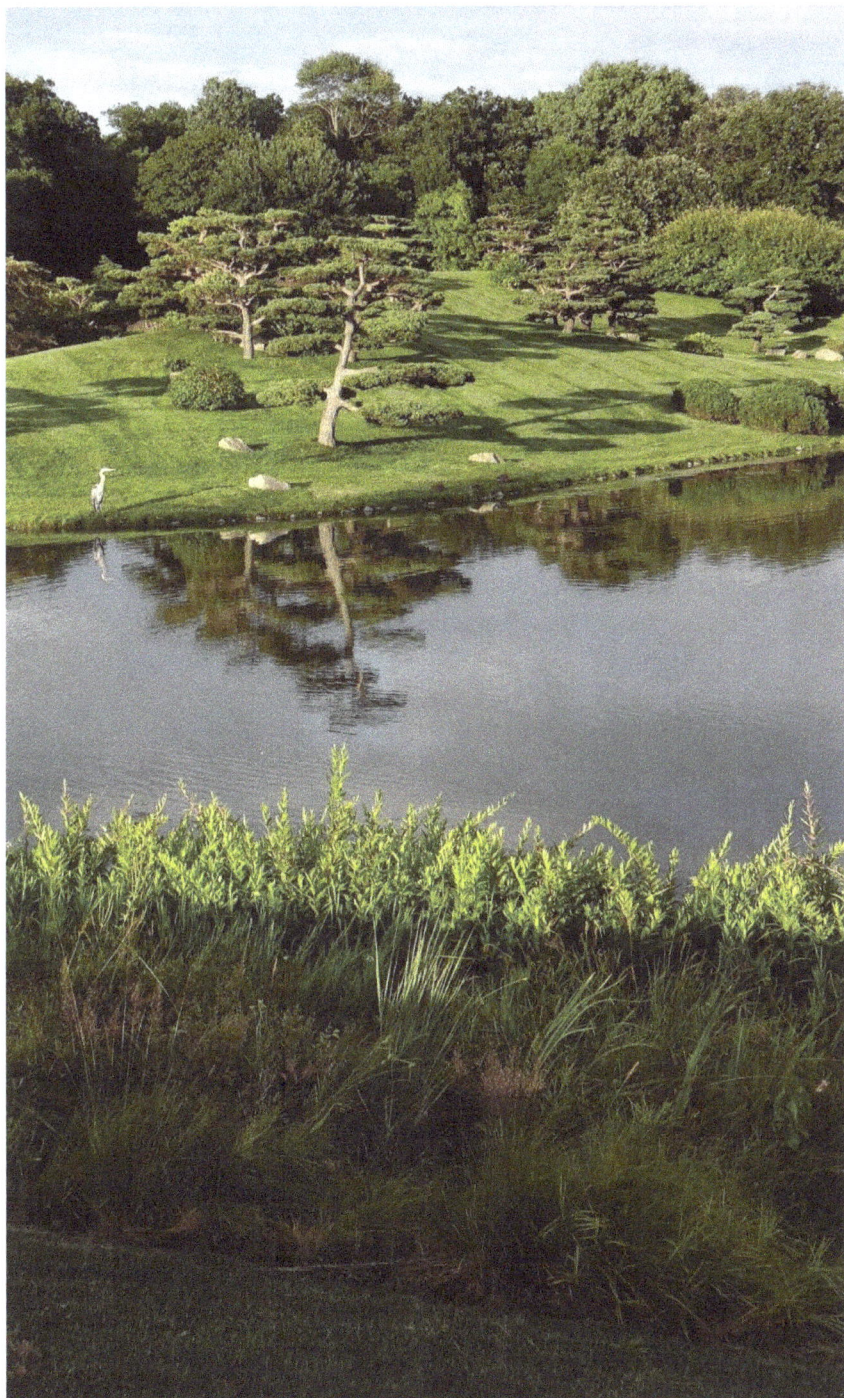

"Have a good night's sleep to be happy.
Be happy to get a good night's sleep."

—*Dr. Venkata L Buddharaju*

SECTION 1

Chapter 1
Sleep Basics

Nature plays a vital role in shaping sleep patterns for all creatures on Earth. Birds, butterflies, fish, mammals, and even plants respond to light-dark cycles. Humans can't ignore nature's long-established sleep patterns, either. Before digital technology, humans awoke with sunrise, spent most of their time in nature, and rested after sunset. They maintained natural circadian rhythms.

While other species have continued to follow natural patterns, human curiosity has caused us to seek improvements to our lives. We have invented comforts like artificial light, televisions, computers, and cell phones. But exposure to natural light at the right time of day is crucial to maintaining a proper circadian rhythm. Unfortunately, we are now constantly exposed to artificial light and technology inputs throughout the day and night, making it difficult for many of us to fall asleep.

Before the industrial and tech revolutions and excess artificial light, people used to go to bed early after sunset and rise early with sunrise, keeping in sync with their natural circadian rhythm (clock). The newer generation of people is increasingly spending late nights watching TV shows, games, movies, screens (computers, cell phones), and other light-emitting devices. They are going to bed late and waking up late after sunrise, a habit that is especially worse on weekends, with some people even sleeping until late mornings. This habit throws the circadian rhythm out of sync with nature.

What is Sleep?

Sleep is a need-based, reversible, unconscious state induced by changes in the brain. For sleep, people typically assume a supine or sitting posture, become immobile, close their eyes, and experience a decreased response to external stimulation. Brain waves, eye movements, and muscle tone can be very different during the various sleep stages.

Sleep is as natural as drinking when thirsty. We can voluntarily postpone sleep in order to fulfill our daily obligations. We can yawn, move around, walk, talk, and even drink caffeinated beverages to fight our need for sleep. However, we can only postpone so much before nature steps in to take over.

When we sleep well all night, we feel good the next morning and are happy and ready to handle life's daily tasks. On the other hand, we can feel miserable, irritable, and not so happy after a night with fewer sleep hours or poor sleep quality. Ideally, people need a longer, uninterrupted, deep night's sleep to achieve their best during their wake periods.

Without adequate sleep, life becomes miserable, and we risk high blood pressure, stroke, and heart attack. We may also experience poor decision-making and memory, feelings of stress, and be more prone to accidents. Studies have shown that the flu and pneumonia vaccines are more effective when someone sleeps well the night before the vaccination is given.

Sleep and the Brain

Interesting things happen in brain circulation during sleep, especially during deep sleep stages. Accumulated proteins, called amyloids, along with other waste products and toxins are slowly washed away via a system of interconnected structures called the glymphatic system.

Sleep restores the mind and body so that we have the energy we need, can focus during the day, and are capable of cognition. While awake, the brain accumulates several waste products. Scientific studies have shown that sleep clears them. If not cleared, they may lead to neuronal damage and increase the risk of dementia.

A recent Boston University study, published in *Science Journal*, showed that water-like fluid surrounding the brain, called cerebrospinal fluid, pulses like waves during sleep and may help to flush out toxic, memory-impairing proteins from the brain. This study and others have shed light on how sleep disruption and lack of sleep can contribute to memory-impairing conditions like Alzheimer's and age-related memory loss.

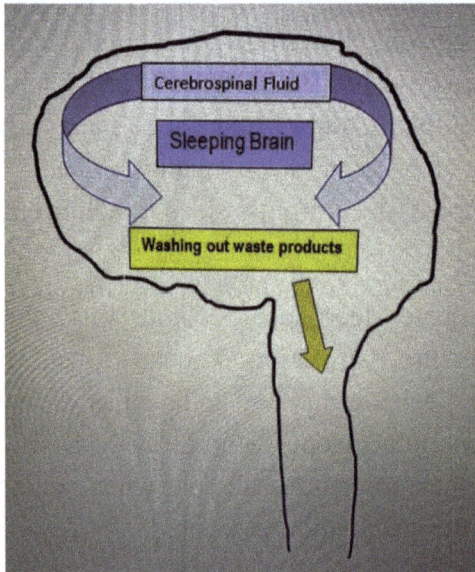

Cerebrospinal Fluid

Sleeping Brain

Washing out waste products

Figure 1: Illustration of how cerebrospinal fluid surrounding the brain washes out the accumulated proteins and toxins during deep sleep to prevent neuronal damage.

Bits and pieces of what we learn during our waking hours are stored in the brain in memory banks during sleep. This is called memory consolidation. It is one of the main reasons that learning happens primarily during deep sleep.

Sleep Stages

Sleep is divided into two main states: non-rapid eye movement sleep (NREM) and REM sleep. NREM is further divided into three stages. Normally, we enter into Stage 1 of sleep 10 to 20 minutes after closing our eyes. It lasts a few minutes and then flows into Stage 2, which is another lighter sleep stage that lasts a little longer than Stage 1. Finally, the deeper sleep, also called **slow wave sleep**, of Stage 3 arrives. This is when most of the body and mind restoration happens. NREM and REM cycles alternate every ninety to one hundred minutes with approximately four to six cycles during a seven-to-nine-hour adult sleep period.

NREM sleep comprises 75 to 80 percent of sleep time. It dominates the first third of the sleep period, with gradual progression from Stage 1, where brain waves will start to slow down to low voltage, and gradually transform into slow wave sleep with higher voltage brain waves in Stage 3. Those who sleep only in lighter sleep stages of 1-2 are not going to get the full benefits of sleep. Patients taking sleeping pills typically spend more time in lighter sleep stages.

REM sleep, which accounts for 20 to 25 percent of sleep, occurs sixty to ninety minutes after sleep onset and dominates the last third of the sleep period. During this stage, brain waves become low voltage and mixed frequency and look like an awake state, but all skeletal muscles relax even more and lose tone to the point of paralysis, except for the heart, diaphragm, and sphincters, which remain active. Your eyes move rapidly during this stage, and dreams typically happen during this stage as well, with the loss of muscle tone preventing you from acting out your dreams. Another very important function that happens is the consolidation of memories and experiences you learned during the day.

Circadian rhythm:

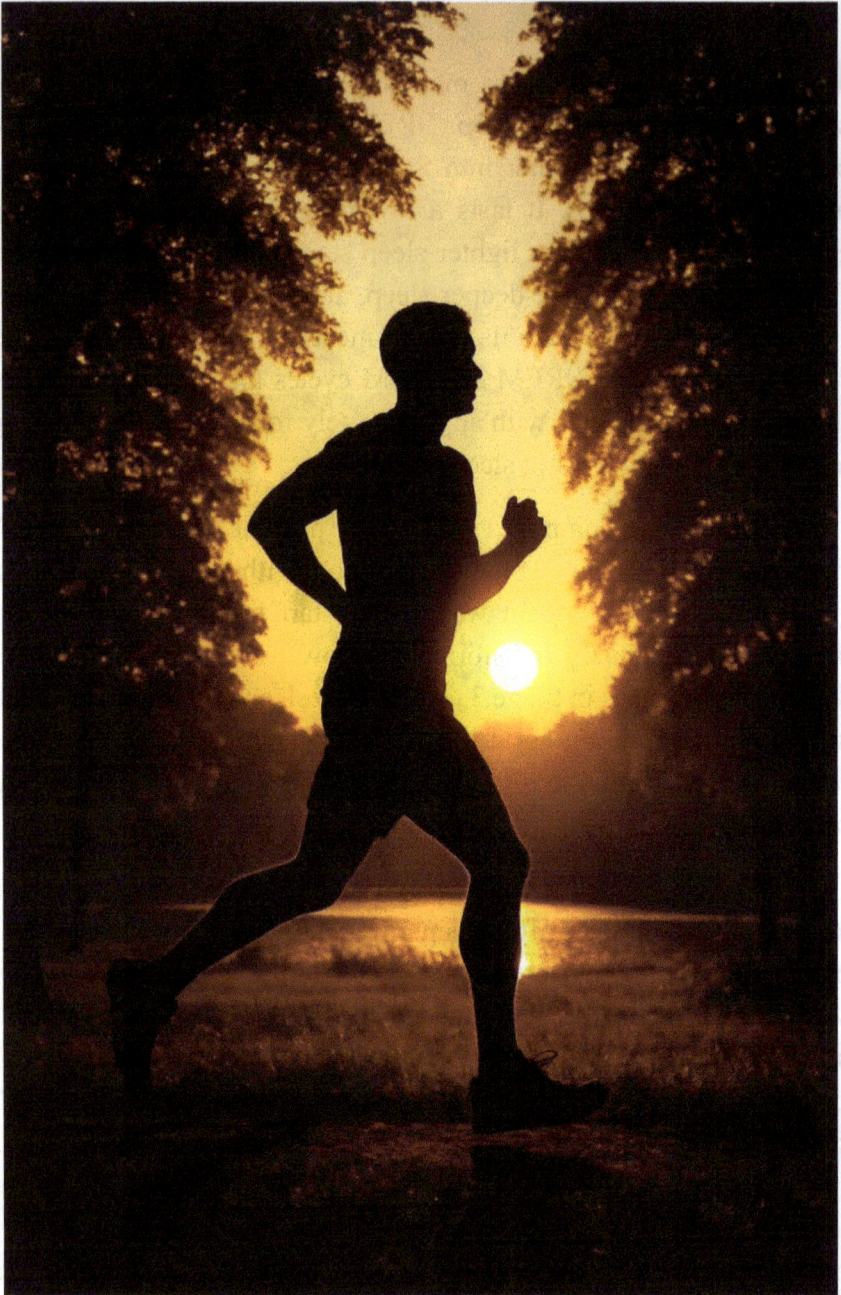

The sleep-wake cycle is tightly regulated by a circadian clock located in the suprachiasmatic nucleus of the hypothalamus in the brain. This is a master switch that controls sleep-wake cycle timings and the body's metabolism, including body temperature. This master clock is influenced by exposure to light and darkness, exercise, eating, and other entraining cues. It also controls the release of melatonin from the pineal gland in darkness, which helps us fall asleep. When we are exposed to too much light, especially when we are supposed to go to bed and sleep after sunset and darkness, melatonin release will be reduced. This is because the eyes send light signals, and the brain is tricked into thinking it is still daylight and therefore cannot go to sleep.

Sleep-Promoting Hormones

Neurochemical messengers released and responsible for sleep and other body functions are as follows:

1. **Melatonin**: A very important sleep hormone released from the brain's pineal gland for sleep initiation, maintaining the sleep-wake cycle, and circadian rhythm. It is also the most common health supplement used today for sleep, with some pros and cons regarding external supplementation versus natural release.

2. **GABA (Gamma-aminobutyric acid)**: An inhibitory neurotransmitter that reduces brain activity, promotes relaxation, and aids sleep.

3. **Adenosine**: Mostly accumulates in the basal forebrain while awake. The longer we are awake, the higher the concentration of adenosine, which promotes sleep. Caffeine counteracts this hormone and keeps one awake. That is why it is not recommended to take coffee or caffeinated beverages at least six to eight hours prior to going to bed, as it interferes with natural sleep.

Wake-Promoting Hormones

1. **Norepinephrine**: Promotes wakefulness.

2. **Orexin**: Promotes wakefulness.

3. **Histamine**: Promotes arousal and wakefulness; that is why when you take an antihistamine, you will feel drowsy.

4. **Cortisol**: A stress hormone that peaks in the morning, helping us wake up and prepare for our day.

Other hormones that control the sleep-wake cycle are serotonin and acetylcholine.

Sleep Duration

Most of the scientific community that studies sleep recommends seven to nine hours of sleep duration for young adults and adults (18-64 years of age) to maintain good health. Older adults (65 and above) still need seven to eight hours of sleep, whereas teenagers (14-17 years) need eight to ten hours of sleep. School-age children (6-13 years) need nine to eleven hours, and preschool-age children (3-5 years) need ten to thirteen hours of sleep.

According to research, people who sleep six hours or less have significantly more lapses in psychomotor vigilance testing. Yet, according to the National Sleep Foundation (NSF), only 10 percent of American adults prioritize sleep over other aspects of life.

I once had a patient who was a cab driver. He worried about losing his driver's license due to his declining health. He worked long hours; his blood pressure and blood sugar were elevated, and he had gained weight eating a high-carb diet and not exercising or sleeping regularly. He drove a cab to pay for his son's college tuition. Workup and evaluation found no sleep disorder. He simply wasn't sleeping the required number of hours. After counseling on sleep, he was able to make changes to his priorities, able to sleep better, and returned to a happy and healthy life.

- **Sleep Deprivation**: Sleep is essential for survival and human health.

Definitions:

- o **Acute**: Less than five hours of uninterrupted sleep.

- o **Chronic Sleep Deprivation (CSD)**: Defined as repeated bouts of insufficient sleep for a long time. Insufficient sleep increases the risk of cardiovascular diseases, premature aging, obesity, poor cognition, and executive function.

According to one study, 25% of the US adult population suffers from CSD. CSD is higher in shift workers and medical professionals.

Chronic sleep deprivation increases the release of the stress hormone cortisol, and people in shift work experience more fatigue, stress, and burnout.

The longer we are awake, the higher the concentration of the sleep-promoting hormone adenosine. The buildup of this hormone throughout the day is why the sleep-wake cycle continues unless interrupted by activity, diet, stress, or health conditions.

Studies have confirmed that good sleep yields better performance, with quality more important than quantity. People need uninterrupted REM sleep to store information.

As mentioned in the introduction, we should spend approximately one-third of our lives sleeping, yet we have gradually reduced sleep duration. According to the CDC, 35 percent of American adults are not getting at least seven hours of sleep on a regular basis. Teenagers need at least eight hours, but a 2006 NSF poll found that 87 percent of high school students in the US get far less.

Let me also reiterate the negative side effects of inadequate sleep: anxiety, depression, suicidal thoughts, obesity, diabetes, hypertension, stroke, heart attack, excessive daytime sleepiness and fatigue, poor concentration, and an increased risk of motor vehicle accidents. These negative side effects are profound, life-altering, and can be life-threatening.

Treatment of these side effects costs billions of dollars annually. As their health declines, sleep-deprived patients wait weeks or months to see doctors and then face the frustration of how to pay for the pills and bills while trying to support their families in a declined state of health. It's a vicious cycle that can be avoided. Let's stay away from those costs and learn to live a happy life with better sleep by incorporating simple lifestyle changes.

Why People Restrict Sleep

Our around-the-clock society demands we stay awake, work, socialize, and entertain. But if the goal is to achieve more, then it is counterproductive to reduce sleep time.

Some have medical conditions that prevent good sleep. Others work nights and have difficulty sleeping and spending time with family, children, and friends.

Poor habits developed from childhood through college will influence sleep periods when starting a new job that demands regular daytime hours. The adaptation can be challenging.

Acute sleep deprivation from attending occasional special events can be quickly recovered with one or two nights of good sleep. Chronic partial sleep deprivation occurs when we regularly reduce sleep time to less than five to six hours. Sleep debt builds up and results in symptoms of sleep deprivation during wake hours.

Nature has strong mechanisms in place to force us to get the sleep we need one way or another. Yet, in the modern world, we try to override these systems all the time. The National Center for Health Statistics found that the average American adult sleeps less than six hours daily. Scientific studies have shown that sleep-deprived individuals suffer from loss of working memory and poor attention.

Psychomotor vigilance testing allows us to measure attention and reaction time to a simple task. The subject is asked to touch the computer screen when numbers pop up. Individuals who slept four to six hours per night had fewer lapses than those who slept four hours or less.

Impact of Sleep on Glucose and Appetite Regulation

With more waking hours, there is more time to make unhealthy choices. Studies have demonstrated that chronic sleep restriction can lead to changes in appetite and increased blood sugar. This is due to the fact that the hormone ghrelin, which tells us when we are hungry and should eat, decreases during sleep. On the other hand, leptin, a hormone that controls our sense of satiety or fullness, increases during sleep. When we get less sleep, the release of these two important hormones is thrown off balance. Hence, more ghrelin is in our systems due to fewer hours of sleep. This can lead to more cravings for high-carbohydrate, sugary, and salty foods, which can result in weight gain and an increased risk of diabetes.

A 2015 Nurses' Health Study linked decreased sleep to an increased risk of diabetes. Studies have also shown that sleep restriction over time can lead to a higher body mass index and obesity in both children and adults.

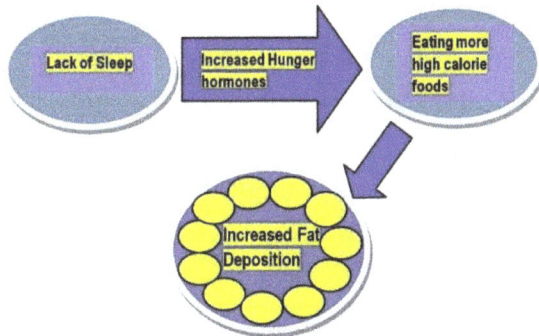

Figure 2: Pictorial description of the Potential Pathway to obesity due to lack of sleep.

Evidence suggests that the hormonal imbalance created by sleep deprivation leads to energy imbalance, weight gain, and obesity. This emphasizes the need for a regular sleep time and duration to curb weight gain and maintain an ideal body weight.

In a recent study of sleep patterns and obesity that was part of a Hispanic Community Health Study, participants between eighteen and sixty-four years old were studied to determine whether there was an association between sleep duration and obesity. The lead author of the study, Dr. Jose S. Loredo of the University of California San Diego School of Medicine, identified an inverse linear association between sleep duration and the prevalence of obesity. Daytime napping was strongly associated with greater obesity. This study was published in the journal *CHEST* in August 2019.

The findings of Dr. Loredo's study suggest that sleep duration and patterns of sleep can have a tremendous effect on a person's weight gain, body mass index, and propensity for obesity. It's my opinion that if a person wants to lose weight, sleep must be part of the plan. In addition to following a strict diet and engaging in regular exercise, sleep quality and duration must be considered. It's clear from the research that if someone wants to lose weight, adequate sleep is necessary. And since regular exercise and a healthy diet promote quality sleep, it becomes clear that one lifestyle change intermingles with the others to help achieve the ideal body weight.

Sleep Restriction and Cognitive Decline

In a study conducted by the National Social Life, Health, and Aging Project (NSHAP), the relationship between sleep and cognition was studied in a group of US adults using **actigraphy**. This is a noninvasive way to monitor rest versus activity with a simple, small device worn over the wrist like a watch. The information gathered by the device is downloaded by researchers for computer analysis. The NSHAP study found that actigraphic sleep disruption—such as waking after sleep onset, sleep fragmentation, percentage of sleep, and wake bouts—were all associated with reduced cognition during daytime hours.

1. **Impact of Sleep Deprivation**: According to the theory of human survival, sleep has a protective and adaptive function and is essential for human survival. Sleep, and especially maintaining a regular sleep-wake schedule, is crucial and essential for maintaining immune defense function against infections.

2. **Nervous System**: Sleep is also important for neural growth and information processing, especially for the growing brain. That is why it is more important for children and young adults to sleep longer than adults because their brains are in an active state of learning. We, and parents, should discourage them from using and staying longer on light-emitting screens. Exposing to light at night causes a shifting of the circadian clock and sleep-wake cycles.

3. **Heart**: Insufficient sleep increases the risk of cardiovascular disease, premature aging, obesity, poor cognition, and executive function. According to a study, 25% of the US adult population suffers from chronic sleep deprivation.

4. **Chronic sleep deprivation** is higher among night shift workers, medical, and other healthcare workers, contributing to higher cortisol levels, stress, fatigue, and burnout. Altering cortisol rhythms and circadian rhythms contribute to difficulty initiating and maintaining sleep.

5. Gastrointestinal System:

During sleep, there is decreased salivation and swallowing, and a general slowdown of the entire system—from the esophagus to the colon—except for the anal sphincter tone, which is preserved to maintain continence of stool. As a result, there is increased acid contact with the esophagus due to reduced peristalsis. Gastric emptying is delayed, especially if you eat late-night meals. It becomes very difficult for digestion and absorption to occur at a time when the system is supposed to be resting (during sleep), compared to the awake state.

Research has shown that poor and inadequate sleep is linked to gastroesophageal reflux disease (GERD), inflammatory bowel disease, constipation, abdominal pain, and even colon cancer due to the increased release of inflammatory cytokines. Lack of sleep can also affect your dietary choices, often leading to cravings for high-calorie and energy-dense foods such as fries and sugary snacks, which are unhealthy and can cause obesity and other health problems.

My message here is: try to sleep and wake at regular times—give or take an hour. Avoid staying up late and don't eat too close to bedtime. If you happen to be out of sync for a few nights, it's no big deal. As soon as you get back on track, the mind and body will fall back into rhythm and adapt.

6. Mind and Psychological Impact:

Sleep is extremely important for regulating emotions. Sleep deprivation can cause anxiety, depression, irritability, and an inability to cope with daily life stresses.

In my own experience, when I've had a good night's sleep, I tend to make better choices—like going for my morning run, eating healthy, making better decisions, and being more productive.

The Best Therapy for Sleep Deprivation

The best therapy for sleep deprivation is to simply sleep more and pay off the sleep debt that was accumulated during the deprivation.

Once in a while, we can stay awake for a longer period of time for important events such as attending a wedding, parties, and socializing with friends and families for long weekends and holidays. Most of this type of short-term sleep loss can be recovered by increasing sleep times after the events. However, for some people, these short-term sleep losses can be more stressful. After acute sleep deprivation of short duration, the majority of people can recover to full alertness with just one or two nights of good sleep. This will restore homeostasis and help them recover from the sleep deprivation. In chronically sleep-restricted situations, however, it is much more difficult to recover. People with chronic sleep deprivation may find it more difficult to stay fully awake, function optimally, or achieve their normal productivity

"If we could give every individual the right amount of nourishment and exercise, not too little and not too much, we would have found the safest way to health."

—Hippocrates

Section 2:
Common Sleep Problems:

Chapter 2
Sleep Disorders

O f the many sleep problems I see in my medical practice, the one that is most common is insomnia. Many patients come to me looking for a prescription for sleeping pills. Their most common complaint is that they are unable to fall asleep after getting into bed. Then, once they finally fall asleep, it's only for a short time. They wake up frequently throughout the night and are exhausted the next day. Nearly 60 million Americans are affected by insomnia each year. It's a major modern health issue with many negative impacts.

In my practice, medication is not my first line of defense. What I find is that most of my patients need only to make small lifestyle changes in order to see big results when it comes to improved sleep. I only prescribe sleeping pills in very rare and difficult situations.

When I'm trying to figure out why a patient can't sleep, I start with some questions. What's your evening routine? What beverages do you consume during the day? What's your morning routine? Tell me about your diet...and so on.

Within a few minutes, I typically start to hear answers that shape my advice to the most exhausted of my patients. I find that the majority of my sleep-deprived patients drink coffee or caffeinated beverages, or take other sleep-inhibiting substances throughout the day and often late into the afternoon. I encourage them to stop this behavior to see if it helps.

Many of my insomnia patients sit at desks all day and don't get much, if any, exercise. I present them with the scientific studies that show a direct relationship between morning exercise and a good night's sleep. I ask them to introduce this healthy behavior into their lives and see if it helps.

Finally, I inquire about their diet. Many of my insomnia patients don't eat a balanced diet. I explain how introducing certain foods can improve their sleep. This is news to most of my patients, but there is a growing body of research on this topic, and I've seen it make a difference in many of my patients' lives. I encourage them to eat more vegetables and fruits, especially kiwifruit, and introduce almonds and walnuts into their diet. I'll explain why this helps with sleep later in this chapter.

My last piece of advice to these patients is to go to sleep and rise at the same time each night and day in order to train their brain. We'll go into all the reasons for these behavioral changes in this chapter, but the results for patients that take this advice are typically very positive. The majority of my patients come back to my office a couple of months later happy and refreshed, telling me that they are sleeping longer hours with minimal interruptions. See? There's no need for sleeping pills in most cases because these simple, natural adjustments to behaviors have corrected the problem. It takes commitment and discipline to make these changes, but the benefits can be life-changing.

In this chapter, we'll take a closer look at some of the most common sleep problems facing people today:

- Insomnia

- Excessive daytime sleepiness

- Obstructive Sleep Apnea

- Circadian sleep disorders

- Shift-work sleep disorders

- Travel-related sleep difficulties

I'll show you simple, natural treatments that can help you stay off sleeping pills and change your sleep patterns from unhealthy to healthy. Among other things, we'll talk about sleep hygiene—what it means and why it's important—as well as negative influences on sleep and how to handle sleep issues during pregnancy.

Insomnia

According to the National Institutes of Health, 30 to 40 percent of adults in the United States claim they have insomnia. Short-term insomnia lasts a few weeks or months and is triggered by life stressors such as a major life event. Chronic insomnia lasts longer and can be related to medical, psychiatric, or pain conditions, poor sleep hygiene, anxiety, depression, or other maladaptive behaviors.

Psychophysiological insomnia is a condition where people are extremely concerned about their inability to sleep and the consequences of sleep loss. They may get better when they sleep away from home due to anxiety related to their bedroom and surroundings.

Associating bedtime and the bedroom environment with sleep is key, reducing time in bed awake to less than twenty minutes. If you are unable to sleep, go to a different place to relax. Avoid exposure to the melatonin-inhibiting blue light of computers and TVs. Watching the clock will only increase anxiety. Practice relaxation therapies prior to bedtime to wind down. Some of the simple tricks that work prior to bedtime are taking a warm bath; sitting down in stillness; performing slow, deep inhalation and exhalation ten times; reading your favorite book; or listening to light, soothing music.

Excessive Daytime Sleepiness

Although some people call this fatigue, **Excessive Daytime Sleepiness** is a real, debilitating health issue. There are a number of sleep disorders that can contribute to this condition, including temporary insomnia due to a life event or more chronic medical conditions such as sleep apnea. Whatever the cause, if the brain doesn't get enough sleep time, it responds with neurochemical triggers that can make you feel tired and sleepy during normal wake hours. The treatment for Excessive Daytime Sleepiness is simple: make lifestyle changes that will help you get optimal uninterrupted sleep at night and treat any underlying medical conditions that are interfering with your sleep regimen.

Obstructive Sleep Apnea

Obstructive Sleep Apnea (OSA) is a condition in which a patient stops or slows down his or her breathing due to a blockage or obstruction at the back of the throat. This is commonly due to the tongue falling back in the throat and blocking the airflow from the nose into the lungs. This condition is commonly seen in obese patients with a body mass index greater than thirty, but it can also be seen in non-obese patients. Once diagnosed in the sleep lab or through a home sleep test, OSA is commonly treated with a CPAP (Continuous Positive Airway Pressure) machine. CPAP stands for continuous positive airway pressure. The machine's pressure is usually set based on the sleep study results. The other ancillary supplies that are used in conjunction with a CPAP machine are a nose mask or pillow, a face mask, tubing, filters, a humidifier, etc. Alternatively, a BiPAP (Bi-level Positive Airway Pressure) mask can be used. This machine with a mask, which is worn over the nose and mouth at night, blows air gently to the back of the throat to open the airway during sleep. This helps patients sleep better and reduces or eliminates their snoring and sleep apnea condition. Along with these medical instruments, patients with OSA should also employ diet and weight loss strategies. Obesity is a risk factor for sleep apnea. Non-obese patients can also get this condition if the upper airway is anatomically narrow and crowded.

Circadian Sleep Disorders (Delayed and Advanced Sleep Phase Syndrome)

I had a male patient who had just finished college and landed a job with a big financial firm. After a few days at his job, he had difficulty waking up and getting to work by 8:00 a.m. He was drowsy and unable to focus because his usual bedtime had been 2:00 a.m., with a wake time between 9:00 a.m. and 10:00 a.m. He was suffering from Delayed Sleep Phase Syndrome, which is common in adolescents. With bright light therapy in the morning, he was able to adjust to his new sleep schedule.

Similarly, night-shift employees are susceptible to sleep difficulties because of the mismatch between their internal brain clock and their work schedule. Night-shift employees also are at an increased risk for social and family problems and drug and alcohol addiction. Daytime sleep and planned napping, evening bright light exposure, good sleep hygiene, stress management, exercise, and a balanced diet will all help night-shift employees avoid problems.

Tips for Coping with Night-Shift Work

- Daytime sleep and planned napping

- Evening bright light exposure

- Sleep hygiene practices

- Exercise and balanced diet with fruits and vegetables and stress management as described

Travel across multiple time zones can also cause delayed or advanced sleep phase syndrome due to the temporary misalignment of our internal clock in each new time zone. It takes approximately one day per time zone crossed to adjust to a new destination. Eastward-bound travelers have difficulty going to bed (phase delayed), whereas westward-bound travelers are sleepy in the evening and wake early in the morning (phase advanced). Avoiding morning bright light exposure for three days prior to departing eastward will help adjust to a new time zone.

According to research, frequent jet travel also has health risks such as impaired cognition and an increased risk of cardiovascular disease, diabetes, and cancer.

Section 3:
Natural Methods for Sleep

Chapter 3
Exercise and Sleep

Moderate aerobic exercise helps us fall into a deeper sleep faster and improves blood flow to the brain, building the neural network and improving cognitive abilities. Exercise causes the brain to release **endorphins**, a neurotransmitter that makes you feel happy. As a result, working out for thirty to fifty minutes a day in the morning improves focus and the ability to handle stress better.

Aerobic exercise for 150 minutes a week reduces cognitive decline and improves neuronal function in Alzheimer's patients, likely because the brain releases **serotonin**, another neurotransmitter that improves neural connections. Exercise also increases total sleep time, slow wave (deep) sleep, and REM sleep—all of which support the sleep restoration process. Some of the other general health benefits of exercise are a reduced risk of stroke, heart attack, diabetes, and hypertension.

Incorporating Movement Daily

The most common excuse for not exercising is lack of time. We strive to do things we think matter the most on our daily and never-ending "to do" list. Then, a health crisis brings us back to reality and shows us what the real priorities should be. Unfortunately, some people never get a second chance. Don't make this mistake. Make your health a priority.

In today's world, we live in the fast lane, ignoring the fact that our bodies can only do so much. For some, goals and the drive to achieve them are beyond what they can actually do. I am not saying to lower the bar, just balance work, life, and sleep so you can achieve more. That's right, if you work toward balance, you can actually achieve more than if you run your body into the ground.

I remember walking and bicycling to the market as a child. Now, even when I need to go only a very short distance, I get into my car. Convenience has become the cornerstone of our lives. We can order almost anything with a single click, and it will be delivered to our doorstep. We hardly have a need to move these days. We sit longer hours, barely walk while we're awake, and can't sleep when we go to bed.

Our inventions are designed to bring us comfort and happiness, but many only bring us new problems. We have created a sedentary lifestyle, and it is causing health issues. Living every moment in the best possible health is the key to happiness. If you had all the physical comforts in the world and plenty of money, wouldn't it all be worthless if you were miserable and couldn't sleep?

Timing of Exercise

What is the best time for exercise? On days that I run in the morning, I feel more energetic, handle stress better, and am more focused and productive. When I run in the evening, though, I can go a little longer with less effort. And as long as I don't run too close to bedtime, it doesn't interfere with my sleep.

Morning Exercise and Weight Loss

For those who would like to lose a few pounds as part of their diet plan, it's a good idea to work out in the morning. According to a recent study from the University of California at Irvine published in *The Journal of Cell Metabolism* in April 2019, morning exercise is best because the metabolic rate is high, causing greater utilization of carbohydrates, ketones, fats, and amino acids. This, in turn, maximizes metabolic and energy benefits and helps to lose weight. Additionally, working out too close to bedtime may prevent sleep as

catecholamine, a wake-promoting hormone, is released.

Cultivate a daily ten, twenty, or thirty-minute exercise routine. Choose an activity you like that you can do at home. People with arthritis or leg problems or who are obese should try swimming for less impact. Incorporate weight lifting or a pressure-load activity twice a week to keep muscles toned. Once you develop a routine, stick to it at least five days a week and make it enjoyable by listening to your favorite music.

Our minds are most alert and active in the morning after waking up from good sleep. Then, slowly, our mind gets warmed up as more information starts pouring in from all directions. We begin multitasking, working on projects or other things that we need to take care of. Sometime in the afternoon—around 2:00 or 3:00 p.m.—our natural circadian clock dips us down. We feel drowsy, a bit sleepy. In some parts of the world, like my home country of India, businesses close in the afternoon to allow for some rest. Businesses reopen again in the early evening, when our circadian clock is most active. It dips back down again, so we can move into a sleep state, after sunset. The eastern part of the world seems to follow the natural pattern of the circadian clock, allowing people to take twenty or thirty-minute afternoon naps to refresh themselves. The western world, by contrast, works all day without a nap break.

Cultivate a daily routine. When you get out of bed, exercise for at least twenty or thirty minutes—even ten minutes of exercise has benefits. Make a habit of doing an activity that you like. For example, walk, go up and down steps, bicycle, do pushups or abdominal curls—whatever you enjoy, do it for twenty or thirty minutes. If time is an issue, you can do these exercises at home, so you don't have to spend time driving to a gym. Remember, some exercise is better than no exercise. Try to do something active each morning.

The simple yet most important lifestyle change I made in my life was setting a regular bedtime around 10:00 p.m. and a regular wake time around 5:00 or 6:00 a.m. This one change has brought me balance and increased productivity. Give it a try and watch your productivity improve.

Morning: Quick Sample Activities

To bring your body and mind into a state of balance, try scheduling the following quick activities into your morning routine when your circadian clock is primed for movement and your metabolism is ready for its morning kickstart.

- Fifty pushups or equivalent of your choice (seven minutes)

- Three yoga steps of your choice with focus on breathing (three minutes)

- Twenty-five seconds standing on a single leg and alternating (two minutes)

- Focused breathing with finger counting with counts of ten (three minutes)

Total time spent: fifteen minutes

Desk Job and Exercise

I once had a patient who was at a desk for eight to twelve hours a day. He suffered from chronic back pain due to poor posture and insomnia, likely from excessive coffee and lack of exercise. One day, he had severe chest pain and was diagnosed with a pulmonary embolism. A blood clot had traveled from his leg to his lung, blocking the transport of oxygen. One of the most common risk factors for this condition is a sedentary lifestyle that allows blood to pool in the legs. My patient has now recovered and no longer takes his health for granted. He now exercises regularly and sleeps soundly.

Depending on the type of work you do, there may be opportunities for you to move or walk throughout the day. For example, if time permits, you could take the stairs to appointments and meetings. The number of steps you choose to take depends on your level of comfort and current physical fitness. I typically take up to three or four floors at a time, and avoid the elevator, if I can. I notice many people waiting at the elevator for a long time. For the time they spend waiting, they could have walked up a whole flight of stairs. People say walking is a waste of time. Is it? When I look at groups of people waiting for the elevator, I notice they are all looking at their phones. They don't even realize how long they are waiting for the elevator. Smartphone addiction distracts us from many priorities in life. Put away your phone and take the stairs. You'll see the health benefits of this small change within a few weeks.

If your work is primarily a desk job in which you spend long hours sitting and looking at computer screens, phone screens, and other devices, you need to carve out time to step away. Stop what you are doing every few hours. Get up and walk around for short distances. Professionals who frequently travel long distances in cars, trucks, or airplanes should do the same. Stop every few hours and do a physical activity. You can take advantage of wearable technology devices to monitor your progress and level of activity.

People with arthritis or leg problems, or people who are obese, often have problems with knee and hip pain. In these cases, they can try swimming, because it is not a weight-bearing activity and puts no pressure on the knees, hips, or ankles.

Try to fit in some weightlifting or pressure-load activities to keep your muscle tone. Do this at least twenty to thirty minutes twice a week. This should help to keep your muscles in condition. If you like riding a bicycle and want to bike to work, this is also a great way to build exercise into a busy morning schedule.

Whatever type of exercise you choose, try to do it consistently. Once you get into a routine, try to stick to the plan and continue the program for at least five days a week.

Sample Exercise Model

If you do thirty minutes of exercise five days a week, that equals 150 minutes of moderate activity a week. Over time, this adds up and will improve your health.

Weekdays: Do aerobic exercise (run, swim, walk) for thirty to fifty minutes every other morning. Do isometric exercise for thirty to fifty minutes on the off days to keep your muscles toned. Add five to ten minutes of yoga or meditation after your daily workout.

Weekends: Make up for any days you missed during the week.

Try to avoid long sedentary times such as sitting and lying down. Try to move throughout the day, even at work. Try to take stairs; avoid elevators for trips that are less than three floors. Longer sedentary times are linked to poor sleep, diabetes, heart disease, stroke, dementia, and a shorter life span.

Key Points for Exercise

- Exercise reduces the risk of stroke, heart attack, diabetes, hypertension, dementia, and depression, and helps you get a good night's sleep and maintain a happy mood.

- Ideally, dedicate some time daily, perhaps forty to fifty minutes (or at least ten to twenty minutes), for aerobic activity or some other type of movement. Do this at least three to five times a week.

- Remember to walk or move while you are at work.

- Choose your preferred activity; just make sure to choose something.

- Set small targets and slowly advance as you get comfortable.

Monitor Daily Progress

- Track your daily exercise times until you develop a routine.

- Circle the type of exercise you did and the duration per day.

- Modify and monitor weekly to measure your progress.

- Conduct Aerobic Exercise (AE) in minutes (circle one).

  0   10   20   30   40   50   60

- Conduct Isometric Exercise (IE) in minutes (circle one).

  0   10   20   30   40   50   60

Write the abbreviation for the type of exercise. Then, add the duration of each session (example: AE-30, IE-30).

	Morning	Afternoon	Evening
Monday			
Tuesday			
Wednesday			
Th rsday			
Friday			
Saturday			
Sunday			

You can keep track of your exercise time in the beginning until you get into a routine. After you're in a groove, you don't have to monitor any more.

Exercise and Sleep

Although more research and clinical studies are needed to determine the exact mechanisms of how exercise improves sleep, the majority of the studies I have reviewed show that modest aerobic exercise improves sleep quality and increases slow wave or deep sleep, which is important for sleep health and general wellbeing.

Science has shown that exercise:

- Releases chemicals called endorphins from the brain that make you feel happy. These feel-good hormones are

31

sometimes called a runners high.

- Increases your core body temperature. However, body temperature starts to cool down about one to two hours after exercise, which helps to facilitate the onset of sleep.

- Depends on the individual preference and as to the impact of timing of exercise on their sleep. Some are morning persons, some are evening. However, getting too vigorous a workout close to bedtime may prevent you going into sleep due to accumulation of catecholamine hormones, which contribute to an awake state.

Figure 3: Graphic view of the concept of how exercise improves sleep quality which in turn make you happy so that you can handle daily stress better

Sleep-Building Habits

It's very easy to slip out of good habits that support our health and happiness. You could have a beautiful garden, but if you don't remove the weeds regularly, it will quickly become overgrown and unattractive. The same is true for maintaining good habits and eliminating bad ones from your lifestyle—to keep your mind calm, your body in shape, and to reduce frequent trips to doctors and hospitals.

Let us see which two habits you would like to make a commitment for the next 90 days

At the end of each chapter starting this section I'll give you two habits to build up on and see if you can make a difference in your sleep.

Exercise and Sleep

Habit 1

I will make a commitment to do 150 min of aerobic exercise a week. (50 min 3 times a week or 30 min 5 times a week)

Aerobic exercise includes brisk walking, jogging, running or a treadmill whatever you prefer.

Habit 2

I will try to do the exercise routine as soon as I wake up in the morning time at sunrise so that I can entrain my circadian clock to keep my sleep –wake cycle in shape.

"Eating a balanced diet is the key for good health, sleep, and happiness. Not too much, not too little. Eat when hungry, stop when full."

—Dr. Venkata L Buddharaju

Chapter 4
Diet and Sleep

There is strong scientific data supporting the notion that our sleep patterns and sleep duration influence our eating behavior. Sleep deficiencies are associated with increased hunger for high-calorie and high-carbohydrate foods, which may lead to weight gain and even obesity. Diets that can help sleep initiation and maintenance contain high amounts of melatonin and serotonin. Diets that reduce serotonin levels can cause insomnia.

American adult obesity rates have increased from 33.7 percent to 39.6 percent over the past decade, according to the CDC. Obesity has been linked to sleep apnea, heart disease, hypertension, and diabetes. As a doctor, it is no coincidence to me that obesity rates have skyrocketed at the same time that we have entered a public health sleep crisis. According to the CDC, one third of adults fail to get the recommended seven hours of sleep at night.

Salivary production and gastrointestinal motility decrease during sleep. Gastric acid secretion peaks between 10:00 p.m. and 2:00 a.m. and decreases in the morning hours after awaking. Gastrointestinal motility is lowest during sleep. These normal changes that take place during sleep delay esophageal acid clearance and prolong acid contact with esophageal mucosa in patients with acid reflux. That's one reason why what you eat and when you eat it can influence the quality of your sleep.

Sleep-Encouraging Recipes and Practices

Blue or blackberries, almonds, walnuts, cherries, and kiwifruits can encourage sleep onset and improve sleep duration and quality. These nuts and fruits have a high concentration of the amino acid **tryptophan**, which converts into sleep-promoting melatonin and serotonin—neurotransmitters that encourage and improve sleep. Serotonin is also a 'feel-good' hormone responsible for feelings of happiness.

Below are three recipes that can help you ingest more of these sleep-friendly foods:

- **Cinnamon Turmeric Lemon (or Lime) Water (CTLW).** Drinking the following recipe has curbed my need for coffee, improved my sleep, lessened my fatigue, and kept my mind sharp.

Heat approximately 600 ml of water until it is lukewarm. Add the juice of one lemon (or lime) for taste and Vitamin C. Then, lightly sprinkle the beverage with cinnamon and turmeric powder. Stir until dissolved. Drink this beverage warm on an empty stomach and be prepared to empty your bladder over the next few hours. If you suffer from acid reflux, don't add lemon.

- **Cinnamon and Turmeric.** Both of these spices have been on the forefront of Eastern diets for decades. Because of their flavor and health benefits, they are now gaining popularity in the West as well. Cinnamon has antioxidant properties and can help lower blood sugars. A 2009 study abstract published in the *Journal of Medicinal Food* by Jitomir J and Willoughby DS from the Department of Health, Human Performance Recreation at Baylor University in Texas showed that supplementation of cassia cinnamon facilitates glucose uptake into the cells by improving insulin sensitivity and may attenuate insulin resistance from sleep loss. Turmeric belongs to the ginger family and also has antioxidant and anti-inflammatory properties, with curcumin as the most active compound.

I practice what I preach and I have been drinking it for a decade now.

You might wonder why I'm talking about the CTLW drink in a sleep book—here's my answer.

- CTLW stands for Cinnamon, Turmeric, Lemon or Lime Water.

- **Total quantity:** 600 ml

- **Time of day to drink:** Morning, on an empty stomach

Why in the morning? We often forget to drink the recommended 1 to 2 liters of water per day for an adult. I thought, if you drink at least a third of that amount in the morning, you can always sip the remaining water throughout the day. We're so busy with work, juggling multiple tasks, spending time on the phone, checking emails, talking to people, flying, driving and rarely do we pay attention to drinking enough water, which results in dehydration.

That's exactly why drinking water in the morning can help jumpstart your brain and body for the day. You should make this a habit so you don't forget. The most fascinating thing I discovered is that once you start feeling good from this CTLW ritual, you'll keep coming back to it. It becomes a form of positive reinforcement: "I've got to do this because I felt better yesterday."

Here are four benefits of drinking CTLW for your sleep and overall health:

1. **Hydration:** Studies show that keeping your body and brain well-hydrated helps you fall asleep faster and improves sleep quality. Hydration also helps regulate body temperature, which can impact sleep. Dehydration increases the stress hormone cortisol, making it harder to fall asleep. It's best to hydrate well during the day and avoid drinking too much water close to bedtime to prevent frequent bathroom trips.

2. **Cinnamon:** Cinnamon helps reduce blood sugar levels and has anti-inflammatory properties, both of which can indirectly improve sleep quality.

3. **Turmeric:** Turmeric and its active compound, curcumin, can increase sleep duration and quality due to their anti-inflammatory effects. Studies show that inflammatory mediators and inflammation negatively impact sleep quality.

4. **Lemon or Lime:** These are rich in vitamin C and slightly acidify body fluids. While they may not directly affect sleep, they aid digestion, support overall health, and help reduce the formation of kidney stones. Plus, adding lemon or lime makes the drink more palatable and flavorful; much better than adding sugar.

A few cautions to note:

1. Because this drink contains acid, it may damage tooth enamel (the white part of your teeth). If you have enamel issues,

consider drinking through a straw.

2. Consult your dentist or healthcare provider, especially if you have medical conditions such as heart failure or kidney problems that require water restriction.

3. If you suffer from acid reflux, you may want to avoid adding lemon or lime. Always consult your physician before introducing CTLW into your daily routine.

- **Soaked Almonds and Walnuts**. The following recipe helped me to eat more nuts, which, as I mentioned earlier, can help your body create sleep-encouraging chemicals. I find it easier and tastier to eat soaked nuts rather than dry nuts.

Soak a handful of raw almonds and walnuts in drinking water overnight. The *next morning, remove the* skins of the almonds. Then, eat a few almonds and/or walnuts after or in between drinking the CTLW.

Other foods rich in tryptophan and serotonin that promote sleep include turkey, chicken, eggs, cheese, tofu, fish (especially salmon), and fruits such as kiwi, bananas, and pineapples, as well as tree nuts like almonds and walnuts. I prefer eating almonds and walnuts soaked overnight in the morning because they become soft and easy to eat.

Sleep-Inhibiting Habits and Substances

While nuts and fruits can help with sleep, other foods, habits, and substances can inhibit the onset of sleep and deprive you of quality sleep. Below is a list of some of the worst sleep-inhibiting foods, habits, and substances.

- **Fatty and oily foods**. Eating fatty or oily foods for dinner or close to bedtime is not conducive to sleep, as your digestive system slows at sunset and can't handle these heavier foods. It is advisable to eat easily digestible, plant-based foods in small quantities in the evening.

- **Late meals**. Eating within a few hours of bedtime is a bad idea unless you are diabetic. As our systems slow in the evening, contractions propel waste to the colon to be eliminated in the morning. Eating close to bedtime interferes with this process and doesn't allow the stomach to rest while we sleep.

- **Caffeine**. Ingesting caffeine in the evening can cause insomnia by counteracting sleep-inducing adenosine, which accumulates in the brain throughout the day during the awake state. When consumed close to bedtime, it delays sleep onset, decreases total sleep time and sleep quality. Caffeine reduces slow wave sleep (deep sleep). Be cautious about drinking coffee or tea (check the caffeine content of your tea) close to bedtime. Different people have different levels of sensitivity to caffeine. Interestingly, increasing caffeine intake over time can lead to an accumulation of adenosine and begin to encourage sleep during the wake period—having the opposite effect that most people hope for when they drink caffeinated beverages. My own experience is that when I cut back or completely stop drinking caffeine, I sleep longer and deeper and feel more refreshed in the morning. If you have sleep problems, cut back or stop drinking coffee—especially in the afternoon, evenings, or close to bedtime.

- **Alcohol**. Acute alcohol intoxication reduces sleep onset time. It can help you sleep deeper in slow-wave sleep during the first half of the night, but the alcohol withdrawal effect in the second half of the night may cause you to be awake and experience increased dreams. With alcohol dependency, total sleep time decreases and becomes more fragmented over time.

- **Tobacco**. Nicotine is a stimulant and can disrupt sleep and increase the risk of sleep apnea. People who quit smoking often experience nicotine withdrawals such as cravings, headaches, and sleepless nights when they give up nicotine.

- **Vaping**. E-cigarettes release nicotine from the liquid after heated by battery. Nicotine stimulates the brain and interferes with sleep, which can cause insomnia. Avoid vaping close to bedtime. There are many unanswered questions about how e-cigarettes will impact health. The issue is being seriously studied by the FDA due to the rapid increase in e-cigarette usage by young people.

- **Marijuana**. Smoking and oral intake of **tetrahydrocannabinol (THC)** reduces time spent in REM sleep, but acute cannabis intake may facilitate sleep and quicker entry into deeper sleep. Withdrawal from cannabis can cause insomnia, vivid dreams, reduced slow-wave sleep, and REM sleep rebound. Long-term studies are needed to fully understand marijuana's impact on sleep, memory, and other bodily functions.

- **Lack of hydration**. A person's daily water requirement varies depending on his or her exposure to sunlight, type of work he or she does, and how much he or she sweats. Listen to your body when it comes to thirst and drink as needed. At a minimum, drinking one to two liters of water per day is essential for maintaining homeostasis. If you have a medical condition that restricts fluid intake, consult your physician for advice on what to drink and how much.

- **Nighttime snacking**. Snacking at night is a bad idea, unless you have diabetes and have to worry about low glucose after you take your insulin. It is best not to eat anything for at least two or three hours prior to bedtime. The reason is that the digestive system goes into sleep mode in the evening. The contractions that propel waste to the colon for elimination in the morning are slowed in the evening as part of your body's natural rhythm. If you start eating at night, too close to bedtime, the food you ingest can interfere with this process. As a result of the evening food intake, the stomach has to fill with acid and try to eliminate the waste at a time when it is supposed to be resting. In other words, you aren't giving the organs in your digestive system time to rest—you're overtaxing them.

Heartburn. For those who suffer from heartburn, which can interfere with sleep, here are some ideas on how to reduce acid reflux-related heartburn:

- Eat small meals throughout the day.

- Avoid eating large meals close to bedtime.

- Don't lie down immediately after meals.

- Eat sitting. Then, walk for a few minutes after meals.

- Sleep with your head and chest elevated forty degrees, left side down.

- Eat whole grains, lean meats, fruits, and vegetables, and limit fried and spicy foods.

- Avoid oranges, lemons, onions, and tomatoes.

Intermittent Fasting (IF) and Type of Diet and Sleep

Research suggests IF may improve sleep quality due to eating on a timed schedule, which coincides with your circadian clock, and in turn helps to maintain your regular sleep-wake cycle.

Few tips:

1. Eat at regular times. Try to eat at least three hours before bedtime to allow for stomach emptying. This also helps to keep your body temperature under control because food digestion and metabolism raise body temperature, which prevents you from getting into deeper sleep.

2. Eat healthy and less oily food at dinner because fat-based food takes longer to empty from the stomach.

3. Don't go to bed hungry because the stress of hunger can raise cortisol levels, which will prevent you from getting to sleep.

4. Always listen to your body and eat when hungry and stop when full to limit what you are eating.

5. A Mediterranean or plant-based diet, which contains fruits, vegetables, nuts and legumes, and healthy fats such as fish with omega-3, has shown better sleep quality and longer sleep due to its anti-inflammatory and antioxidant properties. Fruits such as tart cherry (melatonin) and kiwi, a rich source of serotonin, positively influence sleep.

Sleep-Building Habits

6. I will maintain a daily routine of regular eating times and not disrupt my circadian system.

7. I will eat a sleep-promoting diet and try not to eat late at night or sleep-inhibiting food closer to bedtime.

"A smooth sea never made a skilled sailor."

—Franklin D. Roosevelt

Chapter 5
Stress and Sleep

For the purpose of our discussions in this book, we will define stress as physical and emotional tension related to external or internal events.

Stress can be acute or chronic. Acute stresses are short-lived; our mind and body react, respond, and adapt, and life goes on. On the other hand, chronic stress results from ongoing stressful events that go on for a longer period of time and can affect our physical and mental health.

Over millions of years of biological evolution, nature's successful species have developed stress responses to cope with and adapt to their environment. The human nervous system is no exception. It has evolved in order to survive various threats. Before we began living together in cities, the biggest threat to our survival was from natural predators, like tigers and lions. You have to think fast if you want to outsmart a tiger or lion. This is why one of our natural adaptations is called the **flight-or-fight response**—we have to decide quickly whether we are going to flee when danger strikes or stay and fight. Even today, with no predators threatening us, we still experience our body's flight-or-fight response when confronted with acute stress.

Just as we did years ago when we faced the lions, our bodies release chemicals called epinephrine, norepinephrine, and cortisol. These chemicals trigger glucose sugar production for the quick burst of energy that our muscles need to run. Our heart beats faster to pump blood quickly into our muscles. Our brain is alerted by these chemicals to be more attentive in order to escape the imminent danger. Our other organ systems slow down during these times of stress to keep our body's energy focused on the threat at hand. In these moments, our body and mind prioritize survival—nothing else matters.

The flight-or-fight response has been genetically programmed over millions of years, and it continues to evolve as we evolve. In theory, this stress response should last for a short period of time and should dissipate once the threat has passed.

In today's world, however, we often deal with chronic stress. This means our body stays in a sort of ongoing flight-or-fight mode and continues to release chemicals that it shouldn't release for long periods of time. The consequence of our body's confused state can be high blood pressure, glucose intolerance, sleep difficulties, anxiety, depression, and more. Living in an ongoing flight-or-fight mode is bad for our health. Chronic stress must be addressed to avoid lasting side effects on the mind and body.

Stress is part of life. We can't avoid it. Yet, somehow, we delude ourselves. We go through different stages of life believing that the next stage will be better and less stressful. I hear people say things like, "I will be happy once I complete this task..." or "...after I solve this problem..." or "...when I pass this exam...." In my experience, this notion of "no more stress" in the future is counterproductive. Solutions for one problem can bring new problems. As humans, we are never satisfied. We are constantly scanning for the next threat, the next potential difficulty. We worry and try to avoid these potential threats in order to live a peaceful life. In reality, it is impossible to avoid stressful situations in life. It is much better to learn coping mechanisms that can help us deal with the inevitable stresses that life will throw our way.

When we spend too much time worrying, called **rumination**, our sleep can be disturbed. Worry causes frequent awakening, especially in the early morning hours. Poor quality sleep then results in daytime tiredness and irritability. It becomes a vicious, unhealthy cycle. Therefore, we must learn coping strategies to combat stress and maintain balance in our lives.

Coping Strategies to Reduce Stress

As an Intensive Care Unit physician, I deal with life-threatening emergencies daily and must remain calm and focused on the job. Since daily stressors are ever-present in all our lives, we must learn to control our reactions in order to lead a balanced and healthy life. Unmanaged stress can have a direct impact on our ability to fall asleep and experience quality sleep.

Common emotional reactions to stressors are anxiety and anger, which frequently manifest physically as muscle tension, increased heart rate, sweating, and upset stomach. These reactions can also lead to psychological manifestations such as self-doubt and loss of self-confidence. In turn, these negative emotional states increase our risk of developing high blood pressure or having a heart attack or stroke. As I said earlier, stress can become part of a vicious cycle, destroying our health, peace of mind, and happiness. Needless to say, both the physical and psychological aspects of this cycle can cause sleep difficulties.

Throughout my years as a practicing physician, I have seen a number of techniques help my patients deal with stress. The following methods can help you to stay calm as you deal with problems and stressors. These methods will help you solve issues more effectively and, in turn, get a better night's sleep and stay healthier and happier.

Meditation. Meditative practice improves memory and mental calmness and brings homeostasis to the mind and body. Select the place and posture that best suits you—in a chair, on the floor, or in nature. Focus on the breath coming and going from your nostrils. Every time you complete one deep inhalation and exhalation, count one. Don't judge thoughts that come to mind. Just watch them as a spectator. After a while, your mind will reach a steady state, like calm waters on a lake. That's where your true nature lives. Combining breaths and body movements activates the breathing circuit and vagal nerve. In turn, the parasympathetic nerve fibers counteract the sympathetic overdrive of stress response, calming and slowing the heart. Meditation is safe and is practiced in many parts of the world to overcome suffering, stress, and life's burdens.

Focused breathing. You might call this intentional breathing. To begin, sit up straight and breathe slowly, feeling the air flow in and out as you forget everything for ten to fifteen minutes. Do this at least once a day for better memory and productivity.

Focused breathing with finger counting. Bring the mind to the present moment and focus on your breathing. Take a breath while touching your thumb and index finger. Then, slowly breathe out, removing the thumb from the index finger as you do. Repeat, moving another finger to touch the thumb with each breath. For a count of ten breaths, continue until you complete one cycle. Repeat this process as needed to work through stressful situations.

A common problem described by many of my patients with insomnia is that "My mind races and is too busy with too many thoughts, especially negative ones popping out, and that makes me worry too much, and I cannot go to sleep." One of the solutions for this is to cultivate what is called "Focused breathing and mind watching technique" to bring calmness to the body and mind.

How to Wind Down and Calm Down the Mind and Body Prior to Bedtime:

Mind and thoughts. It's a function of the human brain to produce thoughts constantly; there's nothing much you can do about them. Watch those without reaction, and only pay attention to those that are important and keep others in a watch mode, because they only last for a short period and they are gone and will be replaced by new ones. You will be surprised that your own mind and thoughts change over time.

The mind has a propensity to attach to thoughts, assuming that they come from you. We really don't have a clear answer where thoughts originate and come to our awareness. I personally believe that the mind constantly forms thoughts and brings them to your attention for survival and planning. Some need urgent attention, and others can wait to make decisions at a later time. I believe most of them can be just watched without paying much attention and just being self-aware.

Focused Breathing and mind watching mode (Self-Awareness). You must train and build the skills needed to stay calm and strong to counter the impulses and then reactions to the distractions. First of all, you need to know what the distraction is. Once you identify the distraction, you need to bring in your army of mind power of self-awareness, and now you will automatically become a watcher of those thoughts rather than associate with them. The mind can trick you into believing that these thoughts are yours to own, and you are responsible to act and be part of them. However, you have to be careful and identify which ones you need to act on and which ones you can ignore and keep watching so that you don't get involved and get emotional to react.

If you need help, always go back to the technique of focused breathing and mind watching mode and pay full attention to air flow in and out of your nose, bringing your attention to the present moment, which will calm you down. Stay focused. Cut off the noise at all costs. Don't answer any phone calls that you don't recognize. Do not answer any phone calls that you don't like to talk to. Do not respond to messages that potentially distract you and drain your energy away from the task that you are focused on. "Don't feel bad what happened in the past, don't worry about the future, do what is best now."

Walks in nature. It is difficult to enjoy the natural light of the sun, moon, and stars if you are indoors working all day or live in the middle of a big city. Find time to walk in nature. Bring yourself fully into the present moment as you experience the natural world. Feel your feet as you are walking. Listen to the breeze as it rustles leaves on a tree. Hear the birds' songs and feel connected with nature. Disconnect from technology and spend time thinking and exploring your talents while you are in nature. It will rejuvenate you.

Positive thinking. Your mindset is powerful. It can shape your life. A positive mindset can help you through rough patches. When things go wrong, try to remain confident that life will get better. Think of your worldly problems drifting by like passing clouds. In your darker hours, remember that the light will always shine again. Find opportunities to learn from adversity because you cannot avoid it.

Avoid bad habits. Do not surrender to high-risk behaviors such as excessive drinking, drugs, and smoking. They might give you momentary relief from stress, but they will ultimately impact your health and well-being negatively.

Don't ignore your problems. Recognize that some suffering is necessary for human growth. If we are open to it, adversity can provide opportunities to learn and improve. Master the art of addressing problems directly and dealing with stress effectively and naturally through the techniques outlined in this chapter. Work to overcome your problems with patience and persistence. This will help you develop stress resistance and attain mental calmness, health, happiness, and better sleep throughout your life.

I know it can be difficult to practice these methods in the middle of a crisis, but it is worth the effort to learn. Intentionally applying these simple practices will help your mind lead your body to a calmer place, so you can pick the best strategy or option to resolve the problems you are facing.

As I mentioned earlier in this chapter, I face many challenges throughout my work day as a critical care physician. I deal with life-threatening emergencies and perform life-saving procedures on my patients. One moment, I might be intubating a patient with an endotracheal tube because he has stopped breathing. The next moment, I might be connecting a patient to a ventilator for breathing support or putting an intravenous catheter into his or her heart for an infusion of medications or fluids. No matter what I am asked to do, I must remain calm. The lives of my patients depend on it. Staying focused while performing these procedures is a necessity for patient safety and optimal outcomes. Every hour of the day, I must make timely, critical medical decisions in life-or-death situations.

I also understand my patients' stress and the stress experienced by their families. I know it's very challenging to take care of sick patients. I feel a sense of deep fulfillment when I am able to help one of my patients, save a life, or comfort people whose family members did not survive despite our best efforts. I try to stay focused on the process of my work, rather than the outcome, which I can't always control. This helps me stay calm and give my best to my patients.

In order to perform to the best of my abilities for my patients, I must walk the talk and practice what I preach. I use the methods listed in this chapter. I follow a healthy daily routine and sleep uninterrupted for at least seven hours a night. I wake at optimal hours aligned with nature's circadian rhythm. I make daily exercise and a healthy diet a priority. Yoga and meditation are part of my weekly rituals. These practices have helped me tremendously in my life, and they can help you, too.

Dealing with Difficult People or Circumstances

Everyone has at least one difficult person or situation in his or her life. Perhaps you have trouble dealing with an ex-spouse, a boss, or a sibling. Maybe you have to deal with a troublesome situation at work, home, or school. Whomever or whatever makes your life difficult, the outcome is anxiety and sometimes anger. Research tells us that how you deal with these negative emotions can have a profound impact on your sleep and your health.

Anxiety is apprehensiveness, worry, or nervousness due to a known trigger or unknown fear. It is manifested as tension, increased heartbeat, sweating, and headaches. There is also doubt and loss of self-confidence whether one can execute the task or resolve a known or unknown threat. Anxiety delays sleep onset and contributes to poor sleep quality.

Anger is an emotional reaction to some trigger associated with a feeling of unhappiness. It may cause physical body sensations, such as an uncomfortable feeling in the stomach or tense arm and leg muscles. Usual triggers for anger are when you perceive that you are treated unfairly, disrespected, and neglected by others.

Some of the unexpected situations that you may face from time to time are a friend or relative not returning your phone calls, social isolation, loss of a job, workplace dissatisfaction, health problems, car accidents, traffic jams, conflict with family or friends, legal troubles, and so forth.

People in such situations can experience anxiety, anger, and hatred. They often express these emotions by shouting and throwing things. These reactions were built into human nature and can happen automatically without self-control.

In the long run, these negative emotional states can upset your peace of mind and happiness and lead to an increased risk of high blood pressure, heart attack, stroke, and sleep difficulties.

As with stress, it is very difficult to eliminate people and factors that contribute to anxiety, anger, or hatred in our lives. That's why we must develop strategies to change how we react to these triggers. We must develop adaptive behaviors. It will require dedication and practice to develop these skills and change our lifestyle and mindset, but I promise you it is worth the effort. We must learn how to deal with life's ambiguities and emotional triggers.

Clinical experience has shown that education and lifestyle changes to improve sleep can be helpful in managing anxiety and stress. Here are some tips I give my patients when life gets stressful:

Learn coping strategies. Stress is part of daily life, especially when your ambitions and goals are set high. Everything comes at a cost. Nothing is free. Learning to cope with stress the right way, rather than through addiction to bad habits, can be challenging but is crucial to your health and well-being.

Work for the sake of work, not accolades. Deeply immerse yourself in the work that you love to do. Don't seek rewards, credit, or attention from your peers. The minute your mind starts seeking recognition, it gets distracted. You stop concentrating on the details of the work you are doing. The quality of your work could suffer as a result.

Avoid shouting and angry arguments. Healthy, constructive feedback is good. But it can make us uncomfortable, no matter how noble the criticizer's intentions. In giving and receiving feedback, avoid raising your voice, shouting, or exchanging bad words or language. When things spiral out of control and civility is lost, both parties can feel threatened. Arguments like this are not good for your relationships, your health, your sleep, or your happiness.

Control your reaction time. Your response and reaction time to negative or uncomfortable comments or situations should be intentional, not reactive. A controlled reaction can dissipate tensions and prevent escalation of the situation. Practice slowing down your reaction time. Practice calm, controlled speech, tone, volume, and body language to handle situations that can otherwise trigger anger or hostility.

If you are religious, pray. Religion benefits those who believe and trust in their God. A number of studies have found that devout people have fewer symptoms of depression and anxiety and a better ability to cope with stress. Some religions believe that suffering is the result of bad karma related to something that happened in a previous life. Believers in these religions accept their suffering, so they can let go of the past. These beliefs help them live happily in the present, instead of constantly asking, "Why is this happening only to me and not others?"

Prayer also helps to reduce pain, suffering, and mental anguish when life hands us difficult situations. Those who strongly believe that God will listen and answer their prayers feel less overwhelmed. This helps them cope and heal.

From time to time, I myself have become angry both at work and at home. The strategy I have used to manage the situation is to simply walk away and give everyone a chance to reassess the situation, calm down, and return with a new mindset about how to solve the issues at hand.

In the heat of the moment, humans, like animals, can feel threatened. Stress hormones skyrocket and can cloud rational thought and behavior. It's better to let your biology calm down before reacting or responding to a perceived threat.

How to Cope with Stressful Situations

When you sense that you are about to break down in an emotional situation, train yourself to stop and take ten breaths. Count each breath by touching your thumb to each of your ten fingers. This will immediately calm you by stimulating the vagus nerve, which counterbalances the sympathetic nerve that is responsible for some of the effects of stress—rapid heartbeat, sweating, muscle tightness, and so on.

Once you feel that your mind and body are under control, your judgment will be clearer, and you can deal more effectively with the threat confronting you. I am not saying to ignore your problems. But if you can master the techniques I describe and learn to face anxiety-producing experiences more effectively right out of the gate, you have a better chance of staying happy and healthy. Over time, these disciplines will help you develop patience, tolerance, and constraint, so that you can return to a state of mental calmness, health, and happiness...and, of course, get a better night's sleep.

Here are the top ten practices that have helped me navigate the rough waters in my life:

1. **Pay attention to a person's body language and facial expression.** This will help you understand how he or she is feeling. Also, using friendly body language yourself—like smiling and making eye contact—can help you build rapport when situations are stressful.

2. **Listen more than you speak.** This way you are learning about the other person's viewpoint and not adding to the problem with the wrong words.

3. **Show concern for others.** Be empathetic.

4. **Let go.** You can't control every situation, so don't try to control any.

5. **Associate with honest, positive people.**

6. **Don't sign up until you read the fine print.** Don't be afraid to say no.

7. **Never take unnecessary risks or intentionally do anything wrong or improper.**

8. **Don't be self-indulgent.** Money and power can bring materialistic fantasies, but not real happiness.

9. **Give more and take less.**

10. **Replace anger with compassion.**

Other Practical Tips and Suggestions to Cope with Daily Stress

Based on my own personal experience and talking and counseling colleagues and patients:

- Turn around negative situations to positive.

- Look for opportunities in failures.

- Don't spend time blaming others.

- Step up to the positive side from the negative and keep going.

- In every situation you are in, by accident or by your own choice, just witness it as is without judging. There is always something to learn from every situation, whether it's a failure or success.

- When it's important, don't postpone; do it now. Keep the flow and pay full attention to the means of the work. Don't rush to finalize anything in life except in an emergency.

- If it's an important project that you need to send an email response for, don't click the send button until you spend at least a few nights of good sleep. It's amazing how your brain gives instructions on how to improve your project. Listen to your brain in the morning after you wake up in a state of calmness; it silently tells you the solutions to the problems.

How to Deal with Daily Stress & Worries?

In my experience, no problem lasts forever. It's an absolute waste of time to worry excessively. A little bit of worry is okay, so that it keeps you focused on problem-solving mode. Everything subsides over time, like passing clouds, good or bad.

You don't want to live like a neurotic, running around looking for problems if you don't have any more to solve for the day.

Here are a few practices that have helped me, each taking about 5 minutes:

1. **Breath stacking with pursed-lip breathing (resistive breathing):** This technique involves taking a deep breath, then taking another small breath on top of it, and another, until your lungs are full. Then, you exhale slowly through pursed lips, resisting the airflow. This can help calm your nervous system and improve lung function.

2. **Candle flame gaze:** Light a candle and focus your gaze on the tip of the flame for 5 minutes. This helps to quiet the mind and improve concentration.

3. **"Fly on the wall" observation:** Observe your mind and body as if you were a neutral observer, like a fly on the wall. Notice thoughts, sensations, and emotions without judgment.

4. **Self-awareness of mind and supreme consciousness:** This practice involves an awareness of your thoughts and a connection to a deeper, more profound sense of self or consciousness beyond your individual thoughts.

How to Control Desires and Temptations

I believe the most important aspect of self-control is paying attention to desires and temptations. I divide this process into three stages:

Stage One: Identification of Temptation Triggers During this stage, you come across various triggers of temptation. For example, after your regular, balanced meal, you suddenly see a nice dessert with lots of sugar. Even though you know eating an additional dessert after your regular meal is really bad for your health, especially if your hemoglobin A1c is high and you're diabetic and taking insulin, your temptation and desire are so intense that you are more likely to surrender to them and eat, even though your stomach is full. That's because your mind is telling you to eat, based on your previous pleasant, dopamine-rich, addictive experience of eating the same dessert in the past.

Stage Two: Acting on the Temptation Trigger Now you are ready to act and go eat the dessert without a second thought. This happens so fast, within a few seconds; for example, you will complete the act and eat the whole dessert. This is the crucial stage where you have an opportunity to stop your trigger by immediately resorting to mindfulness breathing, focusing completely on the breath, despite the intense desire to eat. Try to move away from the stimulus that continues to give suggestions to your mind to complete the act of eating the dessert.

Stage Three: Intense Craving Continues (Consolidation Phase) At this stage, in order to break the craving cycle, you can replace the desired item (the dessert) with a healthy alternative, like a soaked walnut, an almond, or any other healthy fruit without added sugar, to satisfy your cravings. Continue to do meditative breathing for 1 to 2 minutes. Typically, these cravings don't last too long. Once the stimulus is removed and satisfied by eating a healthy fruit or nut, the craving stops for the moment, only to return later after a few hours, or perhaps more frequently for highly addicted individuals, depending on their past experiences. This is also called the consolidation phase, where you're consolidating a different behavior. You must continue to meditate for at least 1 to 2 minutes and breathe, and reward yourself for changing your behavior and for achieving self-control.

Repeat the same cycle for other habits such as smoking, excessive alcohol and drug use, or any other behavior that could cause harm to your physical and mental health. If you like, you can always eat a carrot stick or celery stick, any other healthy fruit or nut, or engage in other healthy habits. You can also always use your meditative breathing technique for 1 to 2 minutes, not necessarily needing to eat a healthy fruit or nut, but engaging your hand and mouth and diverting your mind for a moment.

Daily Practices for Well-being

Practice the following daily, ideally in the morning:

1. I will say no to distractions.

2. I will prioritize my time.

Stress Management

There is no way you can avoid or completely eliminate stress in our lives. That is why I'm talking about how to manage it so it won't impact your health and happiness.

I believe a little bit of anxiety and stress is okay and can even be good, as it helps you pay attention to the details of the work you want to do and do your best. And you can also learn how to cope and manage at the same time.

Chronic stress triggers the release of cortisol and other stress hormones, which in the long run can lead to the release of glucose into the bloodstream, potentially leading to diabetes and other chronic illnesses.

You know it when stress hits you. You get frustrated, angry, want to argue and lash out, and you're unable to share the joy of others, including your family members. You immediately see that you're not in the mood to receive the happiness they want to share with you, including your children, wife, and husband. You also know that you're not with them when they need you. And then you feel guilty for not spending time with joy and happiness with your children, wife, husband, friends, and others. You might also get negative feedback from others, causing them to stop sharing their happy moments with you.

Some of the major reasons why people get stressed out:

1. Work-related issues

2. Finances

3. Hefty goals beyond your reach

4. Relationship-related issues

Now the good news is, you can come back and manage your stress response in a more controlled manner and live a happy, enjoyable life again.

1. Exercise every day.

2. Eat a balanced, healthy diet.

3. Listen to music.

4. Work at a hobby that makes you truly happy and do it.

5. Cut off all distractions, including your phones, computers, and other devices, for at least 30 minutes a day.

6. Socialize with friends and family, and engage in funny and humorous conversations and laugh, laugh, and laugh!

How to wind down the mind

Mindful Awareness Breathing (MAB)

Your mind is constantly producing thoughts, randomly and without your control. That's just its nature. It's probably a misconception to think you can "wind down the mind." The real issue isn't the thoughts themselves, but your reaction and anxiety to them, which can lead to uncomfortable feelings and impact your well-being. The Mindful Awareness Breathing (MAB) technique, when practiced consistently, can help you sleep better, focus on your work, calm down, and reduce anxiety over time, allowing you to deal with difficult life situations more effectively.

Here's how to practice the MAB technique:

Mindful Awareness Breathing (MAB) Technique

1. **Prepare your environment:** Put your phone on silent and move it away to avoid distractions for the next 10 minutes.

Let your family members and friends know you need a quiet atmosphere.

2. **Find a quiet place:** This could be under a tree in a park, in your backyard, or in your house. Sit down and simply be aware that you are sitting.

3. **Focus on your breathing:** Now, begin to watch yourself from an outside perspective, as if your own self or soul is observing your body. Direct your full attention and awareness to your breathing. Notice how the air flows in through your nose and gently lifts your belly and lower ribcage. Feel the sensation of this expansion. You can breathe normally or slightly deeper to truly feel the expansion of your lower ribcage and belly.

4. **Optional breath hold and exhale:** You can also hold your breath briefly for a count of 1, 2, 3, then exhale slowly. As you exhale, feel the air flowing out of your nose and imagine that you are letting go of pressure, like taking the lid off something that was built up inside you. You should gradually notice relaxation and a reduction in tension around your neck and shoulder muscles.

5. **Handling distractions:** If you find yourself distracted by random thoughts, gently redirect your awareness back to your breathing as described above. Let the thoughts remain without reacting to them or assigning any feelings to them. Remember, thoughts arise on their own, without your control, so you don't need to be attached to them. For these 10 minutes of MAB, they are separate from you.

You can practice this MAB technique for at least 10 minutes, twice a day, for it to be effective. You can also do it for 10 breaths whenever you feel stressed during the day or before making a big decision. This will immediately calm your mind, and a calm mind makes better decisions.

For a good night's sleep, I highly recommend doing this MAB after taking a hot shower, just before going to bed. It has definitely helped me sleep better, deeper, and longer. You can call this meditation, self-awareness, or mindfulness, but whatever you call it, it has certainly helped me, and I believe it will help you too. I've found MAB particularly useful when dealing with stressful situations, especially during the COVID-19 pandemic in 2020, as part of my critical care medicine practice in the ICU, where I deal with and manage many life-threatening patient conditions.

Another benefit of MAB is that it helps you stay focused and creative on whatever projects you're working on. It certainly helped me stay focused and creative when developing user-friendly and cost-effective medical devices as part of the company I founded a few years ago (www.acanthusmd.com).

Mindfulness and Self-Awareness

You've probably heard the terms mindfulness and self-awareness many times, especially regarding mindfulness practice. This practice helps bring your attention to the present moment and keeps your mind from wandering into the past or the future.

It can be especially hard to focus on the present moment and pay attention to what you're doing when your mind is busy with so many distractions, and your mental energy is being wasted. I've found it particularly useful to practice self-awareness in daily life. You can be mindful of everything you're doing, every day, every moment, to prevent making mistakes. This is especially important while driving a car; you should only be driving and focusing on the road, not checking emails or text messages. You might wonder why I'm discussing this in a book about sleep. The reason is simple: if you drive with a lot of distractions, the chances of getting into an accident are much higher. This can lead to significant stress, both for you and your car. Your goal is to avoid getting into too much trouble while you're awake because these stressors can spill over and increase your stress hormone levels, keeping you awake when you try to sleep at night.

Artificial intelligence (AI) and sleep

You might wonder why I'm talking about AI in a sleep book. You've likely already heard that AI is pretty much in every space of life since its widespread launch a few years ago, answering questions on internet search engines, identifying buyer choices on commercial platforms, and pervading social media. It's also making significant inroads into healthcare, from listening to human voices and compiling patient interactions to drug discovery and much more. For any new technology, I believe humans should maintain control; otherwise, there's a chance of it potentially taking over our lives in the future.

I believe it's a double-edged sword when it comes to using smartphone screens or any new technology. You should use them only when needed, rather than getting addicted to screens to the point of ruining lives. First of all, you need to take care of yourself, sleep better, be healthy, and use this technology in a smart way, rather than overwhelmingly to the point of impacting your basic needs of sleep and health. The conclusion is that humans should smartly use this new artificial intelligence technology to increase their potential, not the other way around. I think people who invented these new technologies must put checks and balances in place to prevent humans from losing themselves to AI. Otherwise, it will add more stress to humans, causing sleep disruption and health problems such as depression and anxiety, which in turn contribute to a burden on society and ultimately lead to a human existential crisis.

Lastly, a Word on Thoughts – Stress – Sleep.

Many people have a huge misperception when it comes to thoughts and have many questions: "Where do they come from?", "What is the meaning of those?", and "What do I do with those thoughts that are sometimes meaningless, useless, and stupid?"

"How do I deal with the anxiety and stress that these thoughts bring to me, sometimes causing obsession, compulsion, and making me do rituals to ease the tension (Obsessive Compulsive Disorder (OCD))?" Millions of people suffer from these thoughts that make no sense and struggle to discern which ones to ignore and which ones they should pay attention to and respond to.

Science has shown that anxiety and stress can cause sleeplessness, and excess stress hormone cortisol can cause high blood sugar and blood pressure, eventually leading to health problems like insomnia, hypertension, and diabetes.

As I said earlier, thoughts don't mean anything in relation to what kind of person you are. Negative thoughts do not mean bad things will happen; positive thoughts do not mean good things will follow. The world and time move on at their own pace, no matter what you think or what your thoughts are.

Based on my own experience and dealing with many of my patients' sleep problems, my best advice is: don't resist and try to remove thoughts by force. Let thoughts be on their own. Ignore them unless you need to deal with something urgent and important based on facts and your own research.

The more you resist, the more they come right back with more force. However, if you ignore them and tell yourself they are just intrusive thoughts, and let them stay that way, then over time, they diminish in force and leave, and may come back, but they don't bother you much.

When you do MAB, just be aware of the above and keep bringing your attention back to your breathing and the sensation of airflow and the expansion of your ribcage and belly. MAB with deep diaphragmatic breathing stimulates the vagus nerve, which reduces anxiety and brings calmness.

Sleep-Building Habits

1. I will regularly practice MAB at least twice a day for at least 10 minutes, definitely closer to bedtime.

2. I will practice self-awareness and keep my mind in "watch mode" rather than responding or reacting to my thoughts, which I have no control over. Instead, I will let the thoughts be as thoughts rather than resisting them.

"I love sleep. My life has the tendency to fall apart
when I'm awake, you know?"

—*Ernest Hemingway*

Chapter 6
A Word About Sleep Hygiene

Before you can understand good sleep hygiene, you need to become familiar with inadequate sleep hygiene. Inadequate sleep hygiene is basically any behavior or activity that interferes with natural sleep—both wake times and sleep times. Examples of inadequate sleep hygiene are:

- Irregular sleep schedules that vary bedtimes and rise times and allow for excessive daytime napping

- Daily and excessive intake of caffeine or alcohol close to bedtime

- Stress and worry at bedtime

- Too much time spent awake in bed

- Too much exposure to light from TV, computers, or phones close to bedtime

- Lack of a proper sleep environment such as uncomfortable bed surface, temperature, or noise level

General Sleep Hygiene Practices Can Improve Sleep

The following practical tips are useful for daily routines and optimizing sleep duration. Once in a while, if your sleep time or duration is reduced, your sleep drive will get stronger on subsequent nights. This is your body's way of catching up and rectifying the sleep debt. It is a normal response.

Here are some additional practices that can improve the duration and quality of your sleep:

- **Establish regular sleep and wake times.** Try to go to sleep at a regular time each night. This is probably the best habit to keep regular sleep and wake times in sync with your internal sleep-wake clock.

- **Expose yourself to natural sunlight every day** while awake and keep the room dark during bedtime and sleep hours.

- **Limit daytime naps to less than twenty to thirty minutes.**

- **Avoid caffeine and other brain stimulants** close to bedtime.

- **Eat small meals at least one or two hours before bedtime**, and avoid high-fat and spicy foods that can increase acid reflux.

- **Exercise daily**, ideally in the morning or at least three or four hours prior to going to sleep for the night.

- **Go to bed when sleepy and don't spend too much time awake in bed.** If you find that you are not sleepy, go to a different room and engage in some relaxing activities, such as reading a book. Don't expose your body to too much light during this time.

- **Don't engage in emotionally stressful arguments or worries** before bedtime.

- **Keep your bedroom at a cooler temperature** (mid-sixties Fahrenheit range). This temperature promotes sleep.

- **Reduce or avoid noise levels** in the bedroom.

- **Engage in soothing body and mind activities**, such as a warm water bath, meditation, or calm breathing—all will help you to relax and prepare your body and mind for sleep.

Shut Off Those Lights in the Bedroom

Researchers have found that exposure to artificial light, such as TV or bedroom lights, is associated with weight gain in women who sleep less than seven hours at night. Although this was not a controlled study, the results suggest that artificial light exposure is a risk factor for weight gain and obesity. In addition, light exposure during the night can interfere with melatonin release and prevent your body from going into sleep mode.

Neuro-chemical Influences on Sleep

Sleep is affected by the influence of either sleep-promoting or sleep-inhibiting factors. Some of the neurotransmitters responsible for wakefulness are glutamate, dopamine, catecholamines, and histamine. One neurotransmitter that promotes sleep is adenosine, which accumulates in the body during wake periods. The longer you are awake, the higher the concentration of adenosine. Caffeine inhibits the accumulation of adenosine in the body, thereby keeping you awake. Gamma-aminobutyric acid, also referred to as GABA, helps promote sleep by inhibiting arousal hormones. Serotonin, which is a precursor for melatonin, also helps regulate sleep. Tryptophan-rich foods present in various proteins encourage the production of serotonin, which is why people feel sleepy after a meal rich in tryptophan—like turkey at Thanksgiving dinner.

Screen Time and Sleep

Science from the National Sleep Foundation shows that excessive screen time use causes poor sleep, especially looking into screens 1-2 hours before bedtime. Despite these negative sleep effects, half of the population in the US spends time on screens close to bedtime. We are so addicted to smartphone screens that I constantly see people looking into their phone screens while walking on sidewalks and on the streets, amazingly not hitting each other but crossing one another automatically. Typically, I see mostly on my morning run, people looking into their phone on one hand, with a dog or coffee cup on the other hand, constantly looking into the phone screen, sometimes smiling and sometimes angry. I call this "Screen Addiction Syndrome." I believe we are living in the middle of high-level tech and information overload with light and sound exposure to our brains, especially hard if our minds are watching super excited content from screens, contributing to a hyper-arousal state. It is very hard to wind down our minds to a calmer state, which is needed to get into sleep at night.

Sleep-wake cycle disruption and screen time exposure: Much worse is the excess screen time closer to bedtime, which delays and disrupts the natural circadian cycle. Normally, when we wake up in the morning with sunlight, we have higher cortisol levels and are ready for the day's tasks. When it is dark at night, cortisol is lower, and melatonin is naturally released to make us sleepy and maintain natural circadian (sleep-wake) cycles regularly. However, if we watch too many screens and expose ourselves to blue light, the brain thinks it is still daytime and stops the natural release of melatonin, which is our sleep hormone. I am also confused why people take melatonin tablets and still watch light and screens trying to go to sleep. I believe the best habit prior to bedtime is to read a book under ordinary low light and go to sleep when sleepy by turning off the light. This is one habit that helped me to sleep better at night.

Sleep During Pregnancy

Women experience difficulties with sleep during pregnancy due to nausea, vomiting, abdominal discomfort, frequent urination, hormonal changes, fetal movements, and anxiety. Due to these and other pregnancy-related changes, mothers-to-be often have difficulty sleeping at night, which can contribute to daytime sleepiness and low energy.

Snoring, sleep apnea, restless legs, and leg cramps can also be disruptive to sleep during the latter part of pregnancy. There are a number of strategies that can improve sleep during pregnancy.

In addition to your physician's advice, the following general sleep hygiene tips can be helpful to get a better night's sleep when you are pregnant.

- **Get optimal sleep.** Trying to get optimal sleep is not easy during pregnancy. Avoid longer naps to prevent nighttime sleep disruption. Sleep in the left lateral position to improve fetal blood flow. Keep your head at an elevation of forty degrees to reduce acid reflux during sleep.

- **Exercise regularly.** Exercise regularly in any way that is comfortable for you. Try to exercise for at least 30 minutes each day. This will help promote sleep, encourage good circulation, and help you maintain a healthy body weight.

- **Eat a balanced diet.** Eat a balanced diet of carbohydrates, proteins, and fats. Take folate and other supplements, such as iron and other minerals, as prescribed by your physician. This will prevent anemia and leg cramps. Avoid caffeine and spicy food that could cause acid reflux, which you will be especially vulnerable to during pregnancy.

- **Meditate daily.** Practice meditation, focused breathing, yoga, and other relaxation techniques throughout your pregnancy. Not only will they help you sleep, they will keep you calm. Walking in nature and listening to music can also help relax the mind and body.

Sleep disruptions are more likely to occur during pregnancy. Doing daily exercise for at least thirty minutes, eating a balanced diet, meditating, sleeping in the left lateral position, and keeping the head of the bed elevated for acid reflux problems will help mothers-to-be smoothly navigate through their pregnancy and delivery.

Early to Bed and Early to rise, makes a man healthy,
wealthy, and wise"

– Benjamin Franklin

Chapter 7
Time Management and Sleep

Time that has passed can only return as memories. How you spend your time in each twenty-four-hour cycle determines how good you feel and how happy you are. Let's divide waking hours into the following periods: family time, tech time, your time, and work time.

Family Time

It's important to make memories with the people we care about and who care about and love us. I have heard of people who work nonstop until a crisis hits. Then, they regret not spending more time with family and friends. I never thought I'd be that person.

Years ago, I was working longer hours, drinking a lot of coffee, and spending many restless nights with poor sleep. It took a long time for me to realize what was going on and make a change in my life. I cut my work by half and started running in the morning. I made spending time with my wife a priority. I almost completely quit drinking coffee and began sleeping much better. I established much more balance in my life. I can confidently say that today, I am a much happier and healthier person as a result of these lifestyle changes.

Everyone's time will eventually come. We all want our final reflections in life to be about our times with loved ones, rather than our regrets about always working. Children grow up fast if you only see them when they are waking up and getting ready for school and at night when they are asleep. Your spouse and children need your presence, compassion, and love. Achieving great things and having an extensive portfolio will not fulfill your need for human connection.

Adjust how you spend the fixed time you have. It is the only way to get valuable family time to make sweet memories. Your children will remember your efforts and do the same with their offspring. It's your life, and it's moving on in one direction. The priorities change over the course of your life. You may be working very hard many hours a week, whether you are a single entrepreneur, businessman, scientist, academician, or whatever. However, once you get married and have children, your family needs you, and you need them. It's time to reduce your work and balance priorities so that you can enjoy family life, be happy, and make your offspring happy.

Studies have shown that people and academics who work longer hours to reach higher goals and publish more are not happy in their lives. I would imagine it's because they miss little things in life that make them happy. At some point in our life, we all have to slow down, sit down, relax, take a deep breath, and think about what we want to do in our life. There is no perfect solution how to live a balanced life. However, we probably need to constantly adjust our priorities in our fixed wake hours to the things that we really love to do in our life and most importantly, live in the present moment. No matter how much time we spend fulfilling our dreams and passions, don't forget to spend time with your loved ones. What makes you happy at the end is not too much money, but how many people really love you.

Tech Time

I grew up without a cell phone, TV, or computer. Today, people depend on technology in their daily lives. American adults spend an average of eleven hours daily on computer screens watching, reading, and interacting through at least two social media accounts. Now, technology has expanded into every aspect of our lives. For example, in healthcare, robotics are now extensively used for surgeries, electronics are used to help move paralyzed limbs, information technology abounds, and electronic medical records overload doctors, nurses, and other healthcare providers.

Ironically, a new wave of technology, called Artificial Intelligence, uses deep machine learning to help solve the problems we face with information overload. I understand the need for technology. I'm not against it. But as a profession, we feel the negative outcomes of spending too much time looking at computer screens and having less time to listen to our patients.

During my hospital rounds, I encourage my trainee doctors to spend more time with our patients and their families in order to become better doctors. It's time to call for a more balanced approach of technology and its role in our lives. The benefits of technology will be more profound if we can learn to balance our personal and professional tech time with real-world time devoted to human interactions.

Your Time

The importance of daily alone time to organize and prioritize your thoughts cannot be underestimated. Spend at least a few minutes each morning reminding yourself of what needs to be done that day, week, or month. Spend time on life aspirations and getting to know yourself through silence and thought, sensing your greatest talents and skills. Trust yourself, work hard, and dedicate time to achieving small goals one at a time. This will bring tremendous happiness amid the chaos of daily life.

Work Time

Work for basic survival. Work for what you love to do and want to achieve. Work demands continue to increase at an alarming rate, and those who work hard and produce are always in demand and are typically given more work.

Workplace burnout is described by the World Health

Organization as chronic workplace stress that has not been successfully managed. It can occur in any workplace. Focus on the projects that bring the most joy and happiness, control your time, and prioritize jobs.

As city populations grow, people live farther from work and spend more time commuting, which reduces the time spent on exercise, sleep, and with family. In my medical profession, various surveys show that approximately 40 percent of physicians report burnout at work. There are many factors contributing to this burnout. Physicians report that they are working too many hours to manage the overwhelming paperwork and documentation burden that comes with treating patients. A recent study of medical interns and trainees showed that they are spending much more time on computer documentation than at the bedside of their patients. This paper burden impacts our sense of job satisfaction, as most of us pursued medicine in order to help people, not fill out papers.

The medical profession is just one example of an industry with high stress for its workers. In many professions, it is getting hard to balance life and work. But too much work beyond your scheduled hours can become burdensome and encroach on the important time you need for sleep, restful activities, family, exercise, and other life aspirations.

I am sure that other occupations face similar workplace challenges that require attention in understanding their personal, family, and other priorities and how to adapt and balance, so that everyone is happy and gets a good night's sleep.

Tips for Improving Work-Life Balance

Take control of your workload and the time it takes to do the job. Don't be afraid to protect your time for the life that you want to live. Management usually recognizes that happy, well-rested employees are usually more productive.

- **Get a job that inspires you** and improves your sense of accomplishment.

- **Prioritize and balance work and family time** in a flexible way so you can meet the demands and needs of both.

- **Find a hobby that makes you happy.**

- **Keep friends who have positive attitudes** and who are supportive of your goals.

- **Always be positive.** You fail only when you give up, so keep trying.

- **Leave your shoes and work outside** and spend valuable time with your spouse and children.

- **Reduce screen time.** Technology cannot replace human presence.

- **Keep sleep hours between 9:00 p.m. to 10:00 p.m. and 5:00 a.m. to 6:00 a.m.**

- **Create a to-do list** to prioritize tasks and update it daily.

"Music heals and connects cultures and humanity across the globe."

—Dr. Venkata L Buddharaju

Chapter 8
Music and Sleep

Both history and scientific research show that music can be used to improve sleep quality. Listening to your favorite music activates emotional reactions and releases hormones that promote sleep and happiness. By improving mood and reducing stress and anxiety, music promotes relaxation and, thereby, sleep quality.

The more regularly you listen to music, the longer the beneficial effects on sleep. Music has also been shown to reduce symptoms of pain from medical conditions such as fibromyalgia and postoperative pain, which can be associated with poor sleep quality.

Studies have shown that listening to calming music helps to fall asleep faster and improve sleep quality. Music also helps reduce anxiety and has a calming effect due to decreased levels of the stress hormone cortisol, and it also releases dopamine, which is a "feel-good" hormone and can alleviate pain and discomfort.

Music also improves heartbeat regularity and blood pressure. It also improves exercise performance and stamina. No wonder many people, including me, listen to music while running, walking, or doing other aerobic activities.

Adding music to your child's bedtime routine has benefits, too, according to a 2018 study in *Sleep Medicine Reviews* by author J.A. Mindell, et al. Singing lullabies and reading were two of the bedtime routines introduced in the study—both had positive impacts. I'm not sure we even need a study to document this, as we know intuitively from our parents and grandparents that singing calms restless children before bedtime. It is a practice handed down through the generations.

In addition to listening to music, improving your vocal abilities can actually help you sleep. It might seem odd, but it's true. Preliminary studies have shown that strengthening your vocal muscles could help reduce snoring. Singing and snoring are related because they involve many of the same muscles.

I personally feel happy when I sing. For those who enjoy music, I recommend both listening to tunes and singing them to improve sleep, boost happiness, and reduce stress throughout the day.

Sleep-Building Habits

1. I will make a regular habit of listening to my favorite songs or singing or playing my favorite instrument.

2. I will make a habit of listening to mind-calming music, especially in the evening and at bedtime.

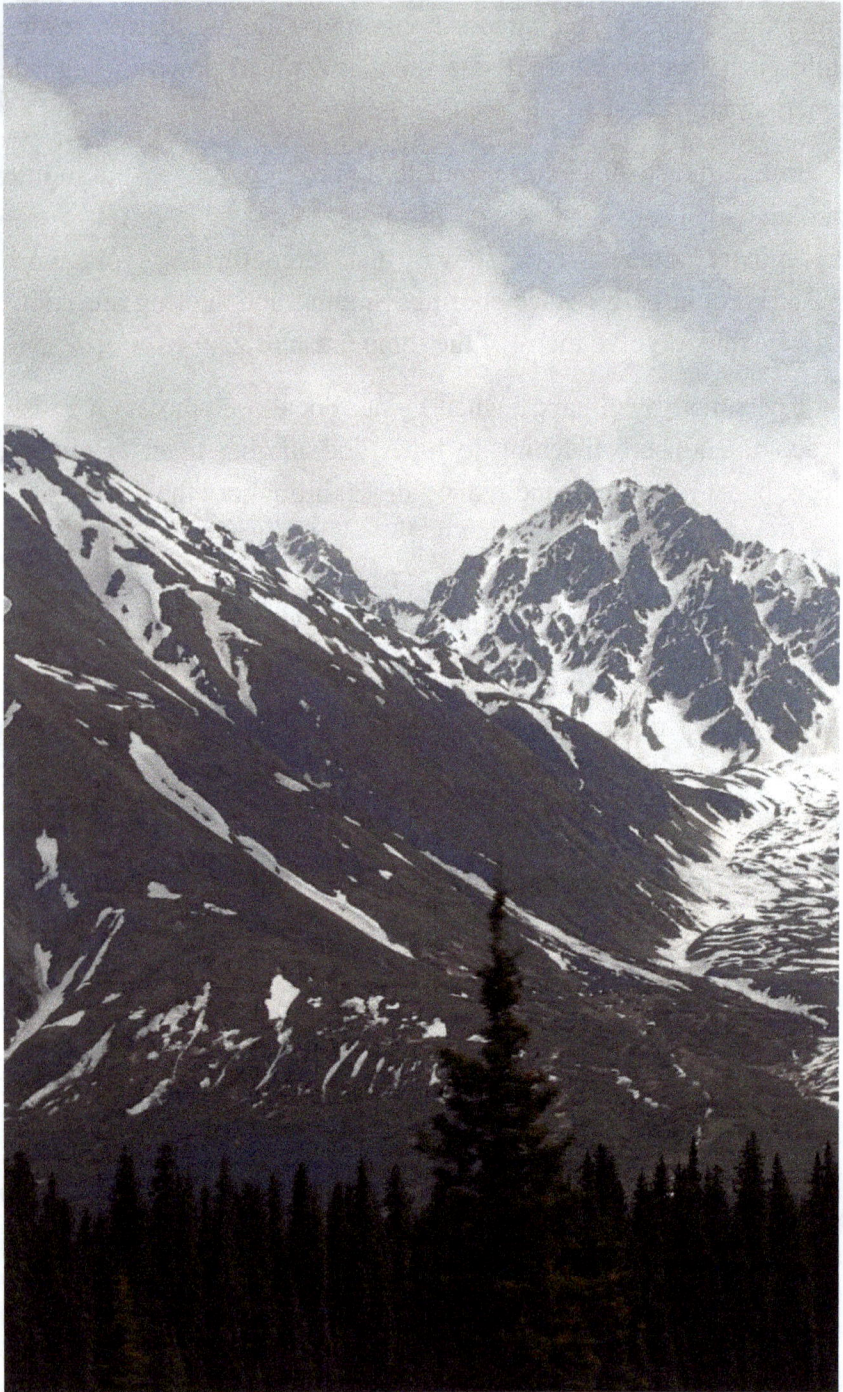

"Living in sync with mother nature's rhythms is essential for sleep, health and happiness"

—Venkata L Buddharaju

Chapter 9
Nature and Sleep

L iving your life connected to nature improves sleep and happiness. Nature calms down the mind and brings peace.

My own personal experience is that after spending time in nature, my mind is calmer, and I am more relaxed and peaceful. Connection with nature helps reduce anxiety and calms down a restless mind. When I jog and run during the morning sunrise, I often imagine that the sun is sending heat and light from millions of miles to the earth, warming the planet, and plants are actively converting that energy to chemical photosynthesis in their leaves. We eat the plant-based food and convert that energy into mechanical movements by moving. Energy is constant but is converting from one form to another.

Nature and Sleep

Nature amazes me. The earth is at a perfect distance from the sun—not too close, not too far—and supports life with just the right amount of light and heat. The earth has maintained rotation around the sun for more than four billion years, keeping the days and nights almost in a balance and allowing us to rest and wake up refreshed to start a new day and do things we love.

Nature has played a vital role in shaping our sleep patterns. Evolved over millions of years, insects, animals, humans, and even plants respond to nature's light-dark cycles, helping us to sleep and wake naturally.

Before digital technology, humans awoke with the sunrise, worked during the daylight, rested at dark, and spent most of their time in nature. Humans maintained natural circadian rhythms and slept optimal hours to live a happy and healthy life.

While the rest of the species on earth continue to move along with nature, humans have invented many ways to "improve" our lives, including artificial light, TV, computers, cell phones, air conditioning, and so much more. Though we have benefited greatly from these inventions, we have also paid a price. For one thing, we are now constantly exposed to light—longer than we would be if we relied only on nature for light. As a result, melatonin, which is produced at a higher level when we are exposed to darkness, is inhibited, making it more difficult to fall asleep. Additionally, the blue light exposure from smartphones can decrease melatonin, a chemical hormone that promotes sleep onset.

Exposure to natural light at the right time of day is crucial to maintaining our brain clocks and ensuring that they work properly. But because of many of our modern conveniences, many of us have difficulty matching our awake state with the morning sunlight and our sleep state with evening twilight.

In nature, the clock genes of various species have evolved differently to maintain a balance and reduce the competition for food and survival of various species who share common ground. If all the species in one area were to awake at the same time and go to sleep at the same time, there would be tremendous competition for food and survival during certain hours of the day. Nature has come up with a system to avoid this issue, so many species can thrive in a specific ecosystem. Isn't nature brilliant?

Let's take a cue from the natural world around us and return to some of the natural practices of our past. Just look around and take note of the balance that most of the species on earth still enjoy while we humans struggle to go to sleep, rest productively, and wake up refreshed. One simple step in this direction is to reduce your exposure to artificial light after sunset. Limiting bright light exposure after sunset helps restore circadian rhythms and sleep patterns.

Exposure to natural sunlight has been associated with improvement in mood, as we know from experiences of people who suffered from winter depression where the exposure of sunlight is limited.

Short Nature Walks

Based on the view of the scientific community, exposure to nature and partaking in "green exercise" has many health benefits. A pilot study of the relationship between health and nature, conducted by C.J. Wood and N. Smyth, showed exposure to nature during childhood, accompanied by exercise, predicted adult nature exposure and green exercises.

The study also showed that connectedness to nature improved patients' ability to deal with stress and was positively associated with lowering heart rate variability during sleep. In conclusion, connectedness to nature is important for adult health, and childhood nature exposure and green exercises are essential to developing this connection.

That's why I recommend that, if time permits, everyone try to spend some time taking short nature walks during the week. Nature assists the human mind and body in its attempts to deal with stress. You can walk, run outdoors, meditate, or do yoga outside, or just sit under a tree or in a park or garden for relaxation. Yes, connecting with nature can lead to better sleep and an overall happier life.

Studies show that spending time in nature, either a short walk, mindful meditation, exercise outdoors in a park or nature, or listening to nature sounds like tree leaves and bird songs, reduces anxiety and has a calming effect on the brain, which improves sleep.

Exposure to natural light at the right times also helps to keep regular sleep-wake cycles.

Sleep-Building Habits

1. I will make it a habit to spend at least 30 minutes outdoors every day. I'll do this by walking, jogging, playing, gardening, or simply sitting under a tree in my backyard or a park. I may also choose to meditate with mindful awareness breathing (MAB) in nature.

2. I will try to expose myself to natural sunlight in the morning to keep my circadian sleep-wake clock in shape.

Sleep Tips

The most important thing you can do to promote sleep at night after sunset is to learn how to get into the winding down mode from the busy workday.

Some of the things you can do to achieve this winding down mode are:

- Stay away from computer screens, video games, TV, phones, and other devices.

- Spend time with family. Don't check emails and phones while eating dinner with family and friends.

- Practice yoga, relaxation, and/or meditation exercises with slow, deep breathing for five to ten minutes.

- Take a warm shower before bedtime.

- Read a favorite book under a readable light; once you feel sleepy, turn off the light and sleep.

- Eat a light dinner at least 3 hours before bedtime.

- Avoid brain-stimulating drinks such as caffeine, especially 8 hours before bedtime.

Epilogue

The requirements of modern life spill over from our wake time into what used to be our sleep time. We sleep less, eat poorly, exercise less, spend more time on our tech devices... and little by little, an unhealthy pattern develops. We can't sleep at night and we're tired during the day. We're unfocused, less productive. We're not as happy as we used to be. We feel more stressed out. We stay up later to try to catch up...and so the cycle continues.

This book, *Sleep Easy with Natural Methods*, was revised with new information added to my previous book, *Better Sleep, Happier Life*, to help people understand the importance of sleep and its relationship to health and happiness. Sleep is a basic human function. It is a requirement for life. Yet, more and more, we treat sleep as if it is a luxury—something we can give up if we need to. This is not the case. Sleep is not a luxury; it is a necessity.

If you are struggling to develop healthy sleep patterns, you might have read other books about sleep. I hope that in this book you found that simple, natural practices can restore rest and rejuvenation in your life. Most of you don't need medication to go to sleep at night or stay asleep. You simply need to make changes to your lifestyle and start to respect the awake and sleep cycle that nature has in place for all of earth's creatures. It takes discipline and practice, but it is very achievable. The sooner you make sleep a priority, the sooner you'll get your life back on track.

I hope you will find practical and useful tips for improving your sleep by reading *Sleep Easy with Natural Methods* and hopefully you will incorporate some of the sleep-building habits into your daily routine to make a difference in your sleep.

I wish you good luck in your journey to better sleep.

Appendix
Good Sleep Hygiene Practices

The following practical tips are useful for optimizing sleep duration:

- **Regular sleep–wake times:** Going to bed at the same time every day is the best way to keep sleep-wake times in sync with your internal clock. Get exposure to natural sunlight daily and keep your room dark during sleep.

- **Limit daytime naps** to thirty minutes.

- **Avoid caffeine and other stimulants** in the evening.

- **Eat small meals** at least one to two hours before bedtime and avoid high-fat and spicy foods that can increase acid reflux and arousal.

- **Exercise** in the morning or at least three hours prior to sleep.

- **Go to bed when sleepy** and don't spend too much time awake in bed. If not sleepy, go to a different room and engage in a relaxing activity such as reading, but don't expose yourself to too much light. Researchers linked exposure to artificial light such as TV or bedroom lights with weight gain in women who sleep less than or more than seven hours.

- **Don't engage in arguments or focus on concerns** before bedtime.

- **Keep the bedroom cool.** Body temperature falls during sleep onset and is lowest in the early morning hours of sleep.

- **Reduce or avoid noise** in the bedroom.

- **Engage in soothing activities** such as warm water baths or meditation to relax the mind.

Self-Care Throughout the Day

Morning

- Drink CTLW (likely a specific beverage mentioned elsewhere in the book, e.g., "Chill-Out Lemon Water").

- Eat a few nuts and some fruit.

- Run or walk outside.

- Briefly stop and rest under a tree. Take a few deep breaths. Watch nature moving the tree leaves and flowers. Listen to the wind and birds and live in the present moment.

- Eat a balanced breakfast—protein, carbohydrate, and a little fat.

Work

1. Focus on what you are doing.

2. Move. Get up every hour or two and walk.

3. Eat a balanced lunch.

4. Take a short afternoon nap, if time permits.

Evening

1. Leave work and enjoy dinner with family.

2. At bedtime, read a book rather than watching TV (to avoid exposure to screen blue light).

Summary of Natural Methods Described in This Book

- **Movement.** Regular exercise will help you sleep, keep you happy, and enable you to handle stress better...so get up and move every day.

- **Good food.** A diet rich in fruits and vegetables with a daily splash of my CTLW drink will improve your sleep.

- **Focused breathing.** Practice focused breathing with finger counting to calm a restless mind during stressful times.

- **Sleep Hygiene.** It's important to have a regular bedtime and wake routine. Avoid online distractions near bedtime.

- **Stress and time management.** How you spend your time during the day and your reaction to stress when you're awake can strongly impact the quality of your sleep at night. This is why time and stress management are so important. Establishing work-life balance, learning to manage stress, and nurturing happy relationships can all improve the quality of your sleep...and your life.

- **Music.** As the great writer and philosopher Kahlil Gibran once said, "Music is the language of the spirit. It opens the secret of life bringing peace, abolishing strife." Listen to music regularly. It has healing powers and will help you relax and sleep better.

- **Nature.** Connect with nature regularly. It has amazing benefits for your sleep and overall health. Nature can calm down a stressed mind.

"Get a good night's sleep and you will be happy.
You will be happy, if you get a good night's sleep."

—Venkata L Buddharaju

Bibliography and Suggested Reading

Introduction and Chapter 1: Sleep Basics

Sleep and the price of Plasticity. Synaptic and cellular homeostasis to memory consolidation and integration. Neuron 2014: 81(1):12-34Tononi G. Cirelli C.

The Glymphatic System – A Beginner's Guide:

Neurochem Res. 2015 Dec; 40(12): 2583–2599.Nadia Aalling Jessen, Anne Sofie Finmann Munk, Iben Lundgaard, and Maiken Nedergaard

Coupled electrophysiological, hemodynamic, and cerebrospinal fluid oscillations in human sleep: Science 01 Nov 2019:Vol. 366, Issue 6465, pages 628-631. Nina E. Fultz, et al

Sleep duration ranges by age groups:

Sleep Health: The Journal of the National Sleep Foundation. February 2017

US Gallup Poll on Sleep: Well-Being December 19, 2013, March 2, 2015 and US gallup poll 2023.

Metabolic consequences of sleep and sleep loss: Sleep Medicine Vol 9, Supplement 1, September 2008, pages S23-S28: Eve Van Cauter, Karine Spiegel, Esra Tasali, Rachel Leproult

Sleep Duration and Cardiovascular disease risk: Epidemiologic and experimental evidence. Sleep Med Clin 2016: 11 (1): 81-89

Sleep Patterns and Obesity: Hispanic Community Health Study: CHEST Vol 156 Issue 2, August 2019, pages 348- 356: Joseph Loredo MD, MPH, et al

Associations of Sleep Characteristics with Cognitive function and decline among older adults: Am J Epidemiol 2019 Jun 1: 188 (6) 1066-1075: McSorley VE, et al

Sleep Dysfunction and Gastrointestinal Diseases: Vikesh Khanijow M.D, et al Gastroenterology & Hepatology Volume 11, Issue 12 December 2015

"Sleep Loss and Emotion: A Systematic Review and Meta-analysis of Over Fifty Years of Experimental Research," Cara Alexis Palmer, PhD et al. *Psychological Bulletin*, published online Dec. 21, 2023.

Chapter 2: Sleep Disorders

Chronic Insomnia, NEJM 2005; 353: 803-810: Michael H Sibler

Cognitive Behavioral Therapy of Insomnia: CHEST 2013; 143 (2) 554-565

The Role of Sleep Hygiene in Promoting Public Health: A Review of Empirical Evidence: Sleep Med Rev 2015 Aug 22: 23-36: Leah A. Irish, Christopher E Kline, et al

Chapter 3: Exercise and Sleep

Exercise and Sleep: Sleep Medicine Reviews: Vol 4 Issue 4, August 2000, pages 387-402: Helen S. Driver, Sheila R. Taylor

The effects of exercise session timing on weight loss and components of energy balance: Midwest exercise trial 2: International Journal of Obesity 09 July 2019: Willis E.A., Creasy, S.A., Honas, J.J, et al

To Investigate the association between sleep and happiness among nurses with different personality traits: A cross–sectional study: The Indian Journal of Occupational therapy: 2019 Vol 51; issue 1 pages 3-7: Sushant Deepak Sarang, et al

Health, happiness, and a good night's sleep: Lancet January 08; 2000: Vol 355 Issue 9198, P155: Sally Hargreaves

Time of Exercise Specifies the Impact on Muscle Metabolic Pathways and Systemic Energy Homeostasis: Vol 30, Issue 1, P92-110. E4, July 02, 2019: Shogo Sato, Astrid Linde Basse, Milena Schonke, Jonas T. Treebak, Juleen R. Zierath, Paolo Sassone-Corsi

Chapter 4: Diet and Sleep

Diet promotes sleep duration and quality: Nutrition Research (2012) 309-319: Katri Peuhkuri, Nora Sihvola, Ritta Korpela

Cinnamon: A Multifaceted Medicinal Plant: Evidence– Based Complementary and Alternative Medicine: Apr 10, 2014. Pasupuleti Visweswara Rao and Siew Hua Gan

Curcumin and its Derivatives: Their Application in Neuropharmacology and Neuroscience in the 21st century: Current Neuropharmacol 2013 Jul; 11(4) 338-378: Wing-Hin Lee, Ching-Yee Loo, et al

Cassia cinnamon for the attenuation of glucose intolerance and insulin resistance resulting from sleep loss: J Med Food 2009 Jun;12(3) 467-72: Jitomir J, Willoughby DS

Chapter 5: Stress and Sleep

Interactions between stress and sleep: from basic research to clinical situations: Sleep Medicine Reviews, Vol 4, No 2, pages 201-219, 2000O. Van Reeth, L Weibel, et al

Chapter 7: Time Management and Sleep

Burnout and satisfaction with work-life balance among US physicians relative to the general US population: Archives Intern Med 2012; 172(18): 1377-1385: Tait D. Shanafelt MD: Sonja Boone, MD; Litjen Tan, PhD, et al

Chapter 8: Music and Sleep

The Music That Helps People Sleep and the Reasons They Believe it Works: A Mixed Methods Analysis of Online Survey

Reports: PLOS: One A Peer-Reviewed, Open Access Journal: PLoS 2018; 13 (11)

Chapter 9: Nature and Sleep

Effect of Natural Sunlight on Sleep Problems and Sleep Quality of the Elderly staying in the nursing home. Holist Nurse Pract 2017 Sept/Oct; 31 (5) 295-302: Duzgun G, Durmaz Akyol A

Circadian Entrainment to the natural light-dark cycle across seasons and the weekend. Current Biology, Vol 27, Issue 4 February 20,2017: Ellen R. Stothard, Andrew W. McHill, et al

The health impact of nature exposure and green exercise across the life course: a pilot study. International Journal of Environmental Health Research Online, March 21, 2019. C. J. Wood &N. Smyth

Sleep Tips

Here's a summary of practical tips for improving sleep:

1. **Lukewarm shower before bed:** Take a warm shower before going to bed to help relax your body and prepare for sleep.

2. **Keep the bedroom cool:** Maintain a slightly cooler bedroom temperature, ideally around 67°F (approximately 19.4°C), as this promotes better sleep.

3. **Avoid screen light exposure at bedtime:** Limit your exposure to light from screens (phones, tablets, computers, TV) close to bedtime, as blue light can interfere with melatonin production and sleep onset.

4. **Avoid Neurostimulants:**

   o Avoid caffeine and other stimulants closer to sleep time.

   o Reduce reliance on TV and other screens.

   o Minimize noise in the bedroom.

5. **GERD and sleep:**

   o Eat a light dinner 3-4 hours prior to bedtime.

   o Avoid spicy and acid-enhancing foods.

   o Try to sleep on your left side down to reduce acid reflux and heartburn.

6. **Bedroom Environment:**

   o Ensure you have a good and comfortable sleeping surface and a pillow.

   o Try to sleep on your left side down.

- o   Maintain an ideal cool temperature of around 67°F.

- o   Remove light-emitting devices such as TVs, smartphones, and other screens from the bedroom.

- o   Instead of screens, read a book.

- o   Go to sleep when you feel sleepy, and turn off all lights in the bedroom except for a low light if needed for walking to the bathroom.

My Daily Routine:

I'm sharing my daily routine, which I try to stick to as closely as possible, with rare exceptions. I have followed this regimen for the past two decades and—knock on wood—my blood pressure, blood sugar levels, and blood panels are all within the normal range for my age.

- **Bedtime:** 10:00–10:30 PM

- **Bedtime reading:** 9:00–10:30 PM

- **Wake-up time:** Between 6:00–7:00 AM

- As soon as I get out of bed, I do 50 pushups.

- I drink my CTLW (600 ml) and eat at least five overnight-soaked almonds and five walnuts, along with fruits.

- **Morning run:** 2–3 miles (about 50 minutes), 3–4 times a week

- **Weightlifting:** 30 minutes, 1–2 times a week

- I drink green tea without sugar or dairy.

- I go to work and take the stairs as much as possible.

- I'm home by 4:00–5:00 PM.

- **Family time / Garden tour:** I spend time with my family and, during the summer, take a walk in my home-grown vegetable garden. (Since I live in the Midwest, I can't do this year-round.)

- **Music time: When in right mood,** I play piano or guitar, practice and sing songs.

- **Nature walks: I spend time walking with my wife especially during summer evenings. Luckily, we have beautiful tree lines, parks around where I live and I have the opportunity to watch beautiful sunsets, listen to birds' songs, and watch blue sky with shinning moon and stars under clouds.**

- **Dinner time:** 6:00–7:00 PM

- **Family time/ work time** 7.00 PM to 10 PM

- **Bedtime and book reading time prior to sleep:** 10-10:30 PM

Best of luck creating your own daily routine that suits you. Just make sure to prioritize one very important thing: a regular sleep-wake cycle. This rhythm is tightly controlled by our genes and natural evolution, and it's key to maintaining good sleep and overall health.

www.ingramcontent.com/pod-product-compliance
Lightning Source LLC
Chambersburg PA
CBHW050528280326
41933CB00011B/1507